HANDBOOK OF THE
BACH FLOWER REMEDIES

ILLUSTRATED

HANDBOOK

of the

Bach Flower
Remedies

Compiled and Edited
by
PHILIP M. CHANCELLOR

THE C. W. DANIEL COMPANY LTD
I CHURCH PATH, SAFFRON WALDEN, ESSEX, CB10 IJP, ENGLAND

This book is respectfully dedicated to Nora Weeks and Victor Bullen, the Jachin and Boaz of the Temple of Healing that Edward Bach brought into being. Together, these dedicated disciples worked for the fulfilment of Dr. Bach's prediction that: "This method of treatment is the medicine of the future, and it will spread through the world." May this wondrous, spiritual, system of healing that Edward Bach discovered and Nora Weeks, together with Victor Bullen propagated, continue to prosper under God's blessing until that day when the Tree of Life shall yield its leaves for the healing of the nations.

CONTENTS

THE COMPOSITE REMEDY

For those unable to treat themselves, treatment can be obtained on application to:—

The Dr. Edward Bach Centre,
Mount Vernon,
Sotwell, Wallingford,
Oxon. OX10 0PZ

Single Stock bottles or the complete set of 38 Remedies can also be obtained from the Centre.

PREFACE

THIS handbook is a compilation of material from many sources. Much of it is taken directly from *The Bach Remedy News Letter* with the kind permission of Nora Weeks who publishes it from the Dr. Edward Bach Healing Centre in England.

The Editor was granted permission to use and adapt the material according to his judgement. It has been freely drawn upon without reference to authorship, except where quotations are indicated. The Editor, however, assumes full responsibility for any errors or contradictory opinions that might appear in the text.

He wishes to thank Miss Weeks not only for her generosity in allowing him to use the material from the *News Letter*, but especially for supplying him with a great amount of unpublished case histories from the records of The Dr. Edward Bach Healing Centre. Although a very busy person, she was never too busy to give of her own good counsel, or to furnish special information when the Editor required it. Indeed, without her wholehearted cooperation, this handbook could never have come into being.

The Editor also acknowledges with thanks, a special debt of gratitude to Rosaleen Spiesse. She most generously gave of her time, not only to make invaluable editorial suggestions, but to painstakingly correct the orthographic errors in the typescript.

This work represents a cooperative effort. It is the hope of those who contributed to that effort that the book will be a fitting tribute to the memory of Dr. Edward Bach, and to the system of healing he discovered and perfected while he was on earth. Since his death thirty-four years ago, the healing work has gone forward and increased. It is aiding suffering humanity throughout almost all of the civilized world, even as he prophesied it would.

PHILIP M. CHANCELLOR

Ixtapan de la Sal
Mexico, 1970

The simple and natural method of healing through the personality, by means of the essence of wild flowers, discovered by Edward Bach, M.B., B.S., M.R.C.S., L.R.C.P., D.P.H. (CAMB.).

———————————

"Let not the simplicity of this method deter you from its use, for you will find the further your researches advance, the greater you will realize the simplicity of all Creation."

"Take no notice of the disease; think only of the outlook on life of the one in distress."

"Final and complete healing will come from within, from the Soul itself, which by His beneficence radiates harmony throughout the personality when allowed to do so."

EDWARD BACH

himself, not the disease, who needs the treatment. It is an absolute exemplar of the old dictum that "there are no diseases, only sick people"! When peace and harmony return to the mind, health and strength will return to the body.

In Dr. Bach's own book, *The Twelve Healers and Other Remedies*, he describes thirty-eight Remedies, one for each of the most common negative states of mind, or moods that afflict mankind. He divided these negative states of mind into seven groups under the following headings: fear; uncertainty; insufficient interest in present circumstances; loneliness; over-sensitivity to influences and ideas; despondency or despair; and over-care for the welfare of others.

Under the heading of FEAR, for instance, there are five Remedies for five different kinds of fear such as: terror, fear of a known cause, fear of an unknown cause, fear of the mind losing control, and fear of other people. As an example, the Remedy for terror or extreme fear (ROCK ROSE) is given when the patient, or those near and dear to him, are seized with sheer terror, when the accident or the illness appears so severe that there is little hope of recovery. The nature of the condition, or the name of the disease makes no difference. If terror is present, then the Remedy for terror is the one which the patient (and his family or friends about him) requires.

The Bach Remedies are absolutely benign in their action; they can never produce an unpleasant reaction under any condition. Therefore they can be safely prescribed and used by anyone, and this was Dr. Bach's intention; that man could bring about his own healing. The Bach Remedies can be taken with any other kind of medicine with absolute safety; there is not the slightest danger of a harmful or conflicting effect to either medicine.

The use of this handbook is ancilliary to *The Twelve Healers and Other Remedies* which gives directions for preparation and dosage. It cannot be too strongly urged that it be read with the latter always at hand, for a thorough understanding of Dr. Bach's book is essential to an understanding of the thirty-eight Flower Remedies. Other books of importance to the student and the practitioner are listed in the bibliography.

PRESCRIBING

PROEM

"The greatest gift that you can give to others is to be happy and hopeful yourself; then you draw them up out of their despondency."

"The action of these remedies is to raise our vibrations and open up our channels for the reception of the Spiritual Self; to flood our natures with the particular virtue we need, and wash out from us the fault that is causing the harm. They are able, like beautiful music or any glorious uplifting thing which gives us inspiration, to raise our very natures, and bring us nearer to our souls and by that very act to bring us peace and relieve our sufferings. They cure, not by attacking the disease, but by flooding our bodies with the beautiful vibrations of our Higher Nature, in the presence of which, disease melts away as snow in the sunshine."

"There is no true healing unless there is a change in outlook, peace of mind, and inner happiness."

EDWARD BACH

CHAPTER I

PRESCRIBING

Prescribing and the Interview

Note: The Editor asked Nora Weeks for her cooperation in outlining the method and procedure which she and Victor Bullen, and without a doubt many, many other Bach practitioners, use in interviewing their patients. She graciously replied with a complete description of her method, and this chapter is written from her letter:

This is a short description of the way in which we prescribe. We do not have a standard list of questions. We feel that it is better to treat each patient as an individual, and in a manner different from any other. This means that each individual must be talked to in a way commensurate with his understanding, his background and his general attitude toward life. The most important thing is to put the patient at his ease; to make him feel that you are his friend and that you sincerely want to help him. Make him feel secure in the fact that he can talk with you about himself in absolute confidence. It is only by talking about himself, without reserve, that you will be able to help him by prescribing the correct Remedy for his condition. Always let him know that he is a fine person, and that he is not the only one in the world who has a similar problem. Assure him sincerely that his difficulties are only temporary, and that his fears are manifesting because he is developing the great courage which is already within him, for fear, after all, is simply a test of courage. Tell him too, that he does have an understanding and a tolerance of others, that his genuine feeling is only overlaid temporarily by impatience and irritability. Assure him again that he is not alone in these emotions, and that the very emotions which are the most troublesome to him can be wholly eliminated. Thus he will gain his freedom. Dr. Bach always used to say: "Tell them they are great! Emphasize their positive qualities! Ask them to think about those and to concentrate on them." Remember, finally and always, that the Spirit is omnipresent, both in your patient and in yourself.

Be sure that each patient receives a warm welcome when he comes into your office. Tell him how glad you are that he has decided to take the Bach Remedies, for they have helped so many people over the past forty years! See that he is comfortably seated, that he is relaxed, and that he is completely at his ease.

You might say something to this effect: "Since you may not know very much about the Bach Flower Remedies, please tell me first about your physical difficulties, and then I will ask you a few questions about yourself." Always remember that the artful practitioner or physician is a good listener! Cultivate this habit and let the patient talk, but be sure to listen attentively! We say this, because in telling us about his physical symptoms, the patient will reveal a great deal about himself, and that is the information that we practitioners are after. He might tell you, all unwittingly, that he is *afraid* the complaint will worsen (MIMULUS), or that he has *lost hope* of ever becoming cured (GORSE). He might say "I get so *impatient* or so *tense* that my work is affected (IMPATIENS)." Indirectly, a patient might remark that he is "really *resentful* about this or that person or condition (WILLOW)." All of these seemingly casual phrases are of the greatest importance to us, especially since they are spontaneous.

The patient's manner of talking is most revealing. How does he talk? Does he talk hurriedly or nervously, or slowly and hesitatingly? Does he speak with great determination, or with the voice of authority; does he whisper with the insecurity of uncertainty and fear? Study the patient's facial expression well, for it reflects his emotions. Is it an expression of worry, or does he frown or blush? Is his smile genuine, or is it forced to cover some deep sorrow or distress? Observe the patient's movements. Does he sit calmly, or does he fidget

with his hands or feet; does he shift his position restlessly in
the chair? All of these details are signs that blazon forth for
those who have eyes to see!

The rule is to listen calmly and to watch closely while the
patient is speaking. Ask a few questions now and then, but
always be careful not to interrupt his talking; wait for a
suitable pause before speaking. You might ask "How long
have you had this trouble? Was there some physical or emotional *shock* connected with it (STAR OF BETHELEHEM)? Was
there a *disappointment*? Is there still a *worry* connected with the
trouble which weighs upon your mind (WHITE CHESTNUT)?"
Take into consideration his age and his general situation,
whether he is married, widowed or single, etc.; does he *dwell
in the past* (HONEYSUCKLE)?

Allow the patient to do most of the talking. Prompt him
when necessary, and ask for a clarification if needed, even
suggest an amplification if the incident seems to warrant it,
or if it appears to have a direct effect upon his emotional
condition. If the patient shows such characteristics as *resentment*, or even the stronger emotions such as *hate*, *envy* or
jealousy (WILLOW), show no sign of surprise or distaste. Assure
the patient that such emotions are the natural products of a
troubled mind that is in a state of discordance; stress that he
will soon be restored to harmony once again, and that he will
find happiness and joy in life. The joy of living is not the
prerogative of a few, but rather it is the *right* of every being
to possess. Show him that negative thoughts poison the system and bring about ill health and unhappiness, and that
such thoughts positively hinder the effectiveness of any treatment. Assure him again of his value as a human being, and of
the importance of the interpersonal relationship between
children of the same Spirit!

Be sure to let him know that *you* are fully aware of his
problems, and that negative thoughts afflict everybody at
some time or other. Some persons have learned to confront
them after having brought their systems and minds into
harmony. That is just what you are going to do with him,
but you will need his cooperation. That is how the Bach

Remedies work. Speak then of his manifold positive qualities; show him the courage that he has displayed in coming this far without giving up hope! Finally, tell him that there is nothing to fear but fear, and that the Remedies which you are going to prescribe for him will help him in every way, mentally and physically. Be positive with your patient; give him every hope. Naturally you cannot guarantee his cure, for only God and his own force of will can do that, but as a human being, and based upon your experience, you can assure him that he will notice a great improvement if he follows faithfully the prescription you have given him. Reassure him that he is not the first person to suffer so, nor will he be the last, but he will certainly be happy to be free from his problems once and for all. Remember that the talk you have with your patient can do very much toward helping him then and there. It will also create a foundation of confidence in you as a practitioner, and in the Remedies as a medicine. Let every patient leave your office feeling better than when he came in. Let this be a cardinal rule of your practice, and your success will be assured!

Prescribing for Oneself

When prescribing Remedies for self-treatment, it is helpful to notice how one reacts to certain circumstances. Observe your own reactions when you are very tired, or in a serious emergency, or when an important decision has to be made, or even when the weather is lowering and gloomy! At such times our defences are down, and our true, one might say, our naked, unadorned, feelings come to the surface, free from self-excusing justifications! (See also reference to self-treatment under "Prescribing for Mental Distress", page 26.)

When we are tired and irritable, and cross with everyone around us, we need IMPATIENS. If we are depressed, and if we seem to find no light or happiness, we need GENTIAN or MUSTARD. Sometimes we may laugh or sing in an effort to be cheerful or in order to appear less tired; that condition calls for AGRIMONY. If we plunge headlong into the bathos of self-pity, we need CHICORY to brace us up. When we seem to lose interest in everything, and to pay no attention to the conversation going on around us, CLEMATIS is indicated. If on the other hand, we feel that life has treated us badly, and that we have too much to do, WILLOW is the Remedy to prescribe.

If we are cool and collected when the kitchen catches fire, we are the VINE type. If we feel frightened of something, we need MIMULUS, and if we become truly terrified, ROCK ROSE.

Let us examine the important question of reaching a decision, for in our reaction lies an answer to our type or character. The Remedies offer the greatest help at such times; let us learn how to avail ourselves of their useful properties. If we seem to be hesitant and indecisive, saying to ourselves "shall I do this or shall I do that" SCLERANTHUS is clearly indicated. If on the other hand we make up our minds immediately, on the basis of a "snap-judgement", and if we feel that others lag behind us in making up *their* minds, we need IMPATIENS, and we may also need further reflection on the matter! If we fear that our decision might not be the right one, take MIMULUS to forget our fear, and to confront the problem head-on. If we have the impulse to ask the opinion of one and all, excepting the opinion of a qualified specialist, we surely need CERATO, and possibly an expert opinion as well!

The matter boils down to this; once our difficulties have been recognized, take the appropriate Remedy, or Remedies, at once. Do not wait until ill or out of sorts! We should welcome the strength these Remedies give us in overcoming our negative states of mind. We may rejoice in the fact that we can remain calm and serene even though we are tired, or have an emergency to meet, a decision to make, or just another grey day to face.

PRESCRIBING FOR PREGNANCY AND CHILDBIRTH

The Remedies are prescribed during the period of pregnancy, labour, and birth, just as they are at any other time, for it is the mood and the outlook, not the condition, which is treated. Actually, the Remedies are particularly useful during these periods. Both pregnancy and childbirth are natural and normal conditions, but they are times when the moods and the states of mind seem to fluctuate more than usual. Since the moods are generally distinctly defined, they can be treated by the prospective mother herself, or by her adviser. A quiet, happy frame of mind is one of the greatest contributing factors toward a painless and easy birth, and today many mothers attend classes to learn how to relax. These lessons will be infinitely easier, and relaxation assured if the prospective mother is helped to control her moods and emotional swings by use of the Remedies.

Some young mothers are nervous and apprehensive as their term approaches. They become tense in mind and in body, even though they were calm and happy up to this point. MIMULUS has proven to be a great help under those conditions; if the fear is very great, ROCK ROSE will help. As an aid to calm the mind, and relax the body, VERVAIN and IMPATIENS may be given. Experience has shown that the RESCUE REMEDY which is described in Chapter 40 has proven to be of great assistance. It is best to start giving it a few days before parturition; mothers to whom the RESCUE REMEDY was given, usually had an easy and gentle birth, and made very rapid recoveries.

A physician who has used the Bach Remedies for many years gave us this account of how he used the Remedies during a confinement:

"Mrs. W., age 33 years, feared that during this, her first pregnancy, she would die at the birth of the child. MIMULUS and ROCK ROSE were prescribed, and these Remedies eliminated the fear and terror. The birth of the child was unusually easy and rapid. Except for some difficulty with the placenta, the condition of the mother and the child was excellent. On the ninth day after the birth, the mother's temperature began to rise, and the following day it rose to 105°F. The patient was restless, and said that she was going to die, and she was very much afraid of death. Her condition was most alarming, and at the request of her family, a specialist was called in consultation. The specialist could not find any physical reason for the high temperature, and he ordered an antistreptococci serum. The next morning her temperature was 104°F and she was still very ill. She remarked: 'If I could get these nervous panics out of my mind, my temperature would go down.' ASPEN was then given, a sip every half an hour to begin with, and when the temperature began to drop, every hour. The temperature began to fall, and at 9 p.m. it was normal, 98.6°F and her pulse was a steady 74. The lochia which had ceased with the rise in temperature returned again, and the patient was once again normal in every way. ASPEN was continued for a long interval, because the patient said that she still had the nervous panics several times a day. She made a complete recovery. She has remained well and without the nervous panics ever since."

PRESCRIBING FOR CHILDREN

The question often arises as to how one should prescribe for children, especially babies who cannot describe their condition. Actually, children suffer from many emotions other than fear and terror, and all of these emotions can cause them great distress and unhappiness. When these difficulties can be overcome in early childhood, the child can be spared much suffering and ill-health in later life.

Children as a rule do not conceal their emotions. Their behaviour in general reflects their feelings. Some babies are fretful, and are only pacified when they are nursed; these are the CHICORY babies who desire that those for whom they care and who care for them *are near them always*. Other babies are really *impatient*, and scream for attention; these, of course, are the IMPATIENS babies. Some babies are happy and gurgling all of the time and they give no trouble unless there really is *something definitely wrong*; these are the AGRIMONY babies. There is the nervous type of baby, who seems to be *frightened* of almost everything; this is the MIMULUS infant. Again, other babies seem to be "old" souls *who live in a world of their own*; they appear to take no notice of anything or anyone; these are the CLEMATIS babies. The CLEMATIS baby almost seems to sleep too much and at times lacks interest even in feeding.

Some children, on the other hand, will try to hide their feelings. They will not tell their parents if they are unhappy at school or if they are bullied by others. Those children who *brood* over their secret difficulties need WHITE CHESTNUT for the *ever recurring thoughts* which go round and round in their heads. Others who appear to be outwardly cheerful, but nevertheless suffer greatly within themselves need AGRIMONY to ease their *mental torture*. Children who hide their *resentment and hatred*, and who try valiantly to overcome such emotions, need WILLOW if they feel that *they have not deserved so great a trial*, or HOLLY if they suffer from thoughts of *jealousy, envy, revenge* or *suspicion*.

Each child, indeed each being, is a distinct personality. In a large family of children, all of whom live under the same conditions and have the same advantages and disadvantages, there will be no two who are alike in temperament. Each will be a unique individual with his own personality. Each in his own way will face life with its shocks and changes, with its adventures and disappointments; each will react differently according to his temperament.

Emotions are very big things in a child's life, and each child battles bravely with them; bravely, because he cannot yet understand why he should have feelings that sadden or depress him instead of making him joyful and happy. He does not understand that he is experiencing the negative characteristics of the fine qualities that he has within him.

Dr. Bach used the treatment of children as the subject of a lecture in which he said:

"We all know how the same illness may effect different people in different ways. If Tommy gets the measles, he may be irritable, Dorothy may be quiet and drowsy. Johnny wants to be petted, little Peter may be all nerves and fearful, while Bobby wants to be alone.

"Now if one disease has such different effects, it is certainly no use treating the disease alone. It is better to treat Tommy, Dorothy, Johnny, Peter and Bobby and get them well; then

goodbye to the measles! What I want to impress upon you is
that it is not the measles which gives the guide to the cure.
It is the way the little one is affected; the mood of the little
one is the most sensitive guide to show what that particular
patient needs.

"Just as moods guide us to the treatment in illness, so also
they may warn us ahead that a complaint is approaching
and enable us to stop the attack. Little Tommy comes home
from school unusually tired, drowsy, or irritable; he may
want to be fussed over or to be left alone. He is 'not quite
himself' as we say. Kind neighbours come in and say: 'Tommy
is sickening for something; you will have to wait.' But why
wait? If Tommy is treated at once according to his mood, he
may soon be turned from 'not quite himself' into 'himself',
and whatever illness was threatened will most likely not
occur, or if it does, it will be so slight as to be hardly noticeable.

"And so with any of us. Before almost all complaints manifest, there is usually a time of 'being not quite fit' or 'a bit run
down'; that is the time to treat the conditions, to get fit, and
to stop things from going further. Prevention is better than
cure, and these Remedies help us in a wonderful way to get
well and to protect ourselves from attack from things
unpleasant."

Since the Bach Remedies are gentle in action and never
give a reaction, and since they are tasteless, they can be given
to babies and children of all ages with perfect confidence. The
dose is the same as for adults, i.e. four drops of the Remedy,
prepared with boiled water for infants, and given either in
the milk formula, in fruit juice, or in water. When the baby is
breast fed, the mother herself can take the Remedy. Normally, four doses of the medicine should be given daily; in
the case of acute illness the dosage may be increased to every
quarter or half hour. This should be continued until the child
shows definite improvement; then the intervals can be longer
until all danger has passed, and the child has recovered.
Remember, the Bach Remedies are never harmful, but that
overdosing does not increase their effectiveness. It is good

practice to continue giving the Remedies four times a day until well after the child has completely recovered.

In severe cases, the Remedies should be changed as the mood of the child changes. For example: the original terror felt by the parents at the onset of a serious condition calls for ROCK ROSE (for both the child and the parents!). As the condition improves, terror becomes anxiety which calls for MIMULUS. Please note that in this case the child is being treated for the mental state of the parents; this is most important, and the mood of the parents is the guide in the case of severe attacks on small babies. Finally when the child has so improved that he himself demonstrates the mood of fretfulness and a desire for attention, the indication has now shifted from the mood of the parents to the mood manifested by the child himself. It is the child's mood that should be treated, and that calls for CHICORY. If the child is in a drowsy state from which it is difficult to arouse him, CLEMATIS is indicated. The child might show temper or impatience, in which case IMPATIENS is the Remedy; should he become demanding, and want the whole family to pay attention to him, that is clearly a case for VINE.

To summarize: change the Remedy as the mood or state of mind changes. If the changes are frequent, prepare small glasses of water with drops of the Remedy required, from which the child can take a sip as needed. Be sure to identify the glasses with a piece of adhesive tape, so you know which remedy is which. The administration of the Remedies is an art. Do it prayerfully, and with loving care. Change the Remedies as a concert organist changes the stops on a great organ to gain the delicate tonal inflections that distinguishes a master of his instrument.

CASE HISTORIES

Girl, age 6. She saw a funeral procession for the first time. Her questions were answered in a simple and forthright manner and the process of death was explained to her. However, she suddenly became obsessed with the fear that her mother would shortly die, and would be taken away from her in a similar procession. She would not let her mother out of her sight. She lost her appetite and had morbid thoughts during the day, and bad dreams at night. RED CHESTNUT was prescribed for her morbid fear regarding her mother; ROCK ROSE for her state of terror. After taking the Remedies for six weeks, she had recovered completely, and was again a happy, normal child.

Girl, age 9. From the time she started to study elementary biology at school, she developed an obsessive fear of dirt. She was always washing her hands to cleanse them of non-existant "dirt". CRAB APPLE was prescribed as a cleansing Remedy. Within one month she had recovered completely from the idea of being unclean.

Girl, age 12. She was very sensitive about spots on her forehead and chin. She was a pretty girl and was very affectionate with her family, but reserved toward strangers. At school she lacked the ability to concentrate. She was dreaming most of the time, and she ignored completely whatever did not interest her. CLEMATIS was prescribed for her daydreams and lack of concentration; CRAB APPLE to cleanse her system of the spots she considered to be so disfiguring. She was also told to add a few drops of CRAB APPLE to some milk and to bathe her face with it every evening. Within three months the spots had disappeared, and once again she became a bright and alert young lady.

Boy, age 9 months. During an air raid in World War II the child was taken into a dark closet by his mother. The noise and the darkness had frightened him greatly, so much so that ever thereafter he could not be left alone in any room, especially in a small room like a bathroom. When he was six years old he was brought to us for treatment. ROCK ROSE was prescribed for terror; MIMULUS for fear of noise and of confined spaces. He took the medicine regularly for three months. At the end of that time he had not only lost his fears, but he became known as the "plucky one" among his schoolmates.

Mrs. E.L.G. wrote to us from Germany as follows: "My

niece recently had a little daughter. The baby is regularly given RESCUE REMEDY which is specially prepared with boiled water. She is as good as gold. If she starts to cry during the night, she is given a few drops of the Remedy in a tea-spoonful of water, and she goes back to sleep immediately. She has never had any of those dreaded crying fits. My niece also puts some of the prepared RESCUE REMEDY on her breasts when she feeds her, so that the baby gets a few drops in her mouth together with the milk. We are very proud of the little girl, and we love her dearly."

PRESCRIBING FOR MENTAL DISTRESS AND EMOTIONAL TENSION

Because of the stress and tension of life today, many people are faced with extreme mental torture. A practitioner is inclined to think first, and sometimes exclusively, of AGRI-MONY alone for these trying and uncomfortable conditions. Actually, each of the thirty-eight states of mind, can, in an extreme form, cause excruciating mental torture. Fortun-ately, the right Remedy at the right time will relieve the tension and the suffering.

There are those people who are tortured ceaselessly by sad or unwanted *thoughts which seem to circle round and round* in their mind, giving them no peace; the Remedy for this is WHITE CHESTNUT. Others suffer from such *depressive anguish* that at times they feel they have reached the limit of human endur-ance; SWEET CHESTNUT is for them. Many persons are often attacked by thoughts of *jealousy, envy, hatred* or *rage*; HOLLY is the remedy for those emotions. Some people fall into such a *dark depression*, without any apparent cause, that there is neither hope nor joy in life, only the black mocking spectre of *hopeless gloom*; MUSTARD is the Remedy for this condition. *Indecision* and *uncertainty* can also cause mental distress, and divert the mind from arriving at a clear resolution; this state calls for SCLERANTHUS. There is the dangerous mood of *deepest despair* which leads to thoughts of *suicide* or of another violent action; CHERRY PLUM can relieve this terrible state. Under certain conditions, *shock* (STAR OF BETHLEHEM), *self-*

reproach (PINE), or *loss of self-confidence* (LARCH) can all cause extreme mental anguish.

The practitioner, as well as the layman who prescribes for himself, should be on the alert for the slightest change of mood. Often, a change of mood presages a more serious condition in the future. It is the red flag of warning. It pays well to heed it!

PRESCRIBING FOR ANIMALS

Many persons have found that the Bach Remedies are most helpful for both animals and plants. This is hardly to be wondered at when we think that both animals and plants have the same temperamental difficulties we have! They too may become frightened, nervous, angry, impatient, dreamy; they may also want to be alone, or to the contrary, they may want continual attention. Each cat or dog, or for that matter every animal and every plant is a definite individual being, and all of us are of the same substance. Therefore it is no wonder that the less evolved creatures and plants also have their own personalities and their own characteristics. If they are closely observed, prescribing for them is not a difficult matter.

CASE HISTORIES

"My Chihuahua was badly injured by a sharp blow on the head and the veterinarian thought that he might lose his eye. I applied the RESCUE REMEDY immediately, and when the bandage was removed four days later, the eye was intact. It has been improving steadily ever since."

"Calves suffering from ringworm responded well to CRAB APPLE and AGRIMONY, the latter because they were tortured by the irritation."

Here is one of Dr. Bach's cases. He saw a man digging a large deep hole in a field nearby where a pony was standing. When Dr. Bach asked what the hole was for, the man replied: "For the pony. She is dying." "Fill up the hole", Dr. Bach said, "the pony will live." He then treated the animal with ROCK ROSE, and within a few days the pony was fit and well again.

"Our cat was hit by an automobile, and both his legs were badly injured. He was in a dreadful state. I gave him ROCK ROSE for the shock; IMPATIENS for the pain and the tension; CRAB APPLE to cleanse his system of any toxins accumulated by the shock. I could only apply them around his head and in his mouth; I dared not touch his legs. The next day I added STAR OF BETHELEHEM to the Remedies and moistened the cushion upon which he was lying with them. After about a week he showed definite signs of recovery, and now even the crushed toes are better."

"My last supply of the RESCUE REMEDY was used on a starling with very good results. The poor bird had been trapped behind my fireplace for about three days, and when I rescued it, it was more dead than alive. I gave him some drops of the RESCUE REMEDY and bathed him with it. He made a marvellous recovery, and flew off to freedom."

"It might interest you to know how the RESCUE REMEDY saved the life of a beautiful peacock. A fox, which killed the peahen, bit the peacock in the neck and pulled out all of his tailfeathers. The bird was truly in a sorry state. I gave some RESCUE REMEDY to the owner of the bird, and he gave it to him in his food. The results were quite remarkable; the peacock made a speedy recovery and will be quite normal again when his tailfeathers grow back."

"Our little Chihuahua had a bad fall and was seriously ill although the veterinarian could not find anything wrong with her. The first dose of the RESCUE REMEDY made a great difference; she perked up amazingly, and within a short time she had recovered completely. The RESCUE REMEDY was also a great help to her when she whelped. I don't know how I could manage without it. Whenever any of the dogs have an injury, I dab some on the sore place, and they get the Remedy by licking themselves. Sometimes they will lick it off my fingers."

Finally, here is a most complete and detailed report from

Mrs. Guy of the Scilly Isles. We are most grateful to her for sending it to us. Mrs. Guy said that the hind leg of her Siamese cat slipped into a deep fryer of hot fat. The poor animal howled with pain and shock. Mrs. Guy reported: "I immediately dashed the RESCUE REMEDY in water over his leg and paw, and smeared it on the side of his mouth where I could. His cries soon ceased. The veterinarian was away from the Island, so I continued to treat the cat with AGRIMONY for the pain and torture, and with CRAB APPLE to cleanse and heal him. I kept putting drops of these Remedies on his paw where the pads had split. As I believe all healing should be gentle, I did not disturb him to examine the damage at this stage; I relied upon the Remedies to heal him. The next morning the paw was badly swollen and the smell was terrible, but he ate and drank well, and rested quietly. By the end of the week, he had torn off the dead skin, and the smell went. The full extent of the injury was then revealed; open wounds and big bare patches, but the paw to which I paid most attention was healed, and it was this paw that had taken the full force of the fat too. All this time his eyes were bright, his bodily functions unimpaired, he had a good appetite, and he showed no signs of shock. His gums had been badly swollen where he had tried to lick the scalding fat off his paw. Now, after six weeks there is only a small wound left and the fur has grown on all the healed parts; this we did not expect. The injured paw is quite normal. Other Remedies were given as required, amongst them strengtheners: CENTAURY, OLIVE and HORNBEAM. When he asked for much attention he was given CHICORY; when he tried to do too much we gave him VERVAIN. MIMULUS was given at first because he was afraid to walk upon the injured foot."

Prescribing for Plants

When treating plants or trees, one must put oneself in their place, and try to imagine how they are feeling. A tree tortured by leaf-curl needs CRAB APPLE as a cleansing remedy as well as AGRIMONY for the torture. A transplanted tree or plant may suffer from shock and this indicates STAR OF BETHLEHEM. If it seems to lack the strength to recover from the transplanting, HORNBEAM or OLIVE should be given. The RESCUE REMEDY has also been found very useful where plants or trees have suffered. A weak or droopy plant could well use the strengthening qualities of CENTAURY, HORNBEAM or OLIVE. Impoverished soil can be sprinkled with the life-giving Remedies of OLIVE, VINE or WILD OAT.

We prepare the Remedies for plants and trees in this way; we fill a one-ounce bottle for the required Remedies with rainwater, and add two drops of each Remedy to the bottle. We put a teaspoon from the bottle into a gallon of rainwater to make a spray for the leaves and the branches, and to water the roots. With trees, be sure to water the ground in a radius equal to the length of the branches in order to reach all of the roots. Actually, here at Mount Vernon we have been almost too busy to do much experimental work with our own garden, but we do have one good case. We had an old apple tree which was covered with "American blight" one summer. We sprayed the trunk and the branches with CRAB APPLE and AGRIMONY, for we felt that the old tree disliked being unclean and felt tortured. We continued to spray for one week, and watered the root area at the same time. The blight soon disappeared, and the tree has never suffered from it again!

CASE HISTORIES

"My nectarine tree, which grew from a nectarine-pip into a lovely straight tree in seven months, suddenly began to wither away and to fail. I found that our cat had gnawed the trunk of the tree two or three inches above the ground. I watered the tree liberally with RESCUE REMEDY and HORNBEAM, and protected it against further harm. When spring came, it literally grew like mad! It had three perfect laterals as well as three or four fruit spurs!"

The following is a rather remarkable report from a friend of the Bach Remedies who was good enough to write us about her experience. "When our cat was ill, his water bowl contained the Remedies we prescribed for him. I used to empty the bowl daily on the same piece of soil in the garden. The year previously, I had planted some cheap Hyacinth bulbs there. When the bulbs came up this year, much to our surprise, all of the bulbs had divided, and instead of three rigid blooms, we had a carpet of first quality blooms that were truly beautiful. The bulbs on either side of the path, which had not received the Remedies, remained single blooms. Since that time whenever I rinse the bottles that contained Remedies, I always pour them on the bulbs alongside the path. Now, they are just coming through, lots of them, and all of them are divided!"

THE PROPHYLACTIC ASPECTS OF THE BACH REMEDIES

A friend of the Bach Remedies, who had used them for many years, wrote to The Dr. Edward Bach Healing Centre. He asked the following question: "How many people think of using the Bach Remedies when they are not ill? Surely they can be used for developing character, developing personality and bringing about a state of super-health?"

The answer to this question is an unequivocal yes; the Bach Remedies most certainly can be used not only to bring about a state of super-health but to maintain it. The Remedies affect the emotions; the emotions affect the physical health of the body; the emotions also serve as an indicator of physical well being, for any emotional imbalance or inharmony is simply a warning of physical conditions to follow. Correct the emotions, and you have forestalled a physical disturbance before it has time to manifest as an illness. Certainly prevention is better than cure, and it is a great misfortune that more people do not pay sufficient attention to the simple but unmistakable emotional signals that reflect a change in the mood or in the state of mind. Were they to do so, much unhappiness and illness could be prevented!

Dr. Bach's gift to the world can be even more appreciated when it is recalled that his method of healing is so safe and so sure that any "compassionate and intelligent" person can use it forthwith, with absolute safety, and with proven results.

Even if an error in prescribing was made, the worst that could happen would be poor results. The wrong Remedy could NOT in any way injure the body, nor cause any reaction whatsoever.

Most certainly prophylactic prevention of illness should be one of the main objectives of Dr. Bach's therapy. Ill-health is the physical manifestation of negative qualities which hinder the development of true character, and the development of character is the reason that we are on this earth. The Remedies are meant for those who truly desire to overcome the obstacles which hinder their progress, and which have to be overcome before such highly desirable qualities such as courage, tolerance, kindness, understanding and peace of mind can be obtained. The obstacles are always present, for it is only by overcoming them that we are able to progress, and as we progress, the obstacles become more and more subtle. By the same law, fortunately, so do the Bach Remedies. On the more practical and material plane of everyday relationships with our fellow men, the Remedies aid in maintaining these even under trying conditions. They sometimes re-establish relationships which have deteriorated, and which have become a source of unhappiness and loneliness.

The person who wrote the letter quoted above went on to say: "I find this kind of prescribing much more difficult than prescribing for someone who is physically ill, for when a person *seems* to be healthy, everything is likely to be played in a minor key."

This is a fair observation. But, when the desire to overcome a negative state of mind is strong enough, whether it is for ourself, or for another who seeks our help, prescribing is not difficult when we discover the emotions responsible for the disharmonious condition. To do this, we must base our assessment on the character as a whole. Our judgement must be absolutely honest and undeceived by either the wishful thinking of justification or the false mask of personality.

Deep within most of us lie traits of character of which we are not proud, and that we would give much to be freed from. Yet, often we lack the courage to bring these unpleasant

traits into the open and face them once and for all. The result
is that over the years we deceive ourselves into believing that
these traits are a fixed part of our immutable nature. We
accept this falsehood, and, rather than trying to correct it,
we bow to what seems to be the inevitable and secretly hope
that it will go away and leave us alone! Be sure it will do
neither; rather, until we control it, it will control us! The
Remedies provide an invaluable help to us under these
conditions. They will give us the strength to bring forth the
undesirable traits, to face them, and once and for all, to free
ourselves from their domination.

There are, in addition to the major traits in our characters
which affect us so strongly, itinerant and passing moods that
influence us also, but to a lesser extent. Sometimes we speak
of "getting out of the wrong side of the bed", and we are
irritated at the breakfast table. Such moods should be dealt
with forthwith! IMPATIENS, for instance, taken immediately
upon awakening should assure a happy breakfast, and a good
start for the day.

By treating an unhappy state of mind when it occurs, ill
health and indeed ill humour can be prevented, for as Dr.
Bach said: "Disease is but the consolidation of a mental
attitude." How obvious this is when one considers the deep
lines formed on the forehead and the sides of the mouth of
the habitual worrier! Or the stiff joints formed in those of
much pride or rigidity of ideas! It is so worthwhile to take
ourselves in hand and to overcome our mental and emotional
difficulties! This is true not only from the standpoint of
physical wellbeing, but from the more important point of our
spiritual advancement! It is so very worthwhile too, to help a
child overcome fear or jealousy or anger, and so enable him
to walk through life happily and with confidence!

Dr. Bach understood this very well when he wrote: "There
are those who need help, if possible even more than those
with bodily pains. There are those who have had only a few,
or perhaps not even one day's illness in their lives, and yet
they suffer greatly mentally, and the anguish of the thought-
pain is often more unbearable than bodily pain."

THE THIRTY-EIGHT REMEDIES

CHAPTER 2

AGRIMONY

Keywords: Mental torture; worry, concealed from others

ON the surface, the AGRIMONY type appears to be very cheerful and carefree. He makes a good companion and he usually has a true sense of humor. It is a pleasure to be with him. For these reasons, it may at first seem difficult to discover the correct Remedy for the person in question. But the AGRIMONY personality wears the mask of carefreeness only superficially, while deep within himself, he is a severely tortured person; the mask only hides a turbulent state of mind. The AGRIMONY type are peace loving people who are distressed by quarrels and arguments. Rather than inflict their troubles upon others, they often make light of their difficulties. At night when they retire, they are often restless, and their churning thoughts are the cause of insomnia and inquietude. During an illness, the AGRIMONY person may well make jokes with those around him or attending him; he is inclined to make light of his discomfort and to appear cheerful and happy. AGRIMONY children are those who can readily forget their worries, cast aside their cares, and resume a cheerful outlook on a moment's notice. The AGRIMONY type is the exact opposite of the HEATHER person, for the latter cannot avoid discussing their symptoms and woes. Both types dislike being alone, but for different reasons. The AGRIMONY person seeks companionship in order to escape from and to forget their worries in pleasant fellowship; the HEATHER type only wants to air his ego-centred personality to anyone who has the patience to listen to him. At times, when they are severely pressed, the AGRIMONY people may resort to alcohol or to drugs in order to dull the mental torture which they are experiencing.

The positive aspect of the AGRIMONY type is reflected in those persons who can truly laugh at their own worries, because they are fully aware of their relative unimportance. They are genuine optimists, and the inveterate peacemakers.

Case Histories

Woman, age 50. She was cheerful, always laughing, and apparently a happy person who could see the funny side of everything. Her husband died one year before she came for treatment, and left her on her own with financial and other worries. During the day she was fully occupied with many interests, but at night she was restless and could not sleep. Her cares and worries descended upon her, and she tossed and turned until the early hours of the morning. This condition had gone on since the death of her husband. Her general health was good, but she felt tired, and she found it difficult to remember details. It was also hard for her to maintain her usual good humor and cheerfulness. AGRIMONY was prescribed for the distress and worry which she so bravely concealed from friends and relatives, as well as for her restlessness and insomnia. OLIVE was added for her exhaustion. Good results were immediate. During the first week she slept seven hours every night, and she awoke relaxed and refreshed. Within six weeks she was again her normal self, and she was well able to confront all of her problems.

Man, age 40. He was a courageous person, but restless, high-strung, and suffered from anxieties. He had many family worries, and he drank heavily to gain relief from his mental torture. AGRIMONY alone was prescribed. After a treatment of two months, he had lost his craving for alcohol and he was able to analyse and resolve his many problems. He had become a normal person again.

Boy, age 9. He had asthma from birth. He was a cheerful and happy child who did not complain during the most severe attacks, and who tried to make the best of his disability. AGRIMONY alone was prescribed. After commencing the treatment, he had one more attack, and after that he was never troubled with asthma again. His recovery was complete.

Woman, age 40, unmarried. She suffered from a rheumatic pain in her upper left arm and shoulder. The pain was so severe that it prevented her from sleeping. When she applied to us for treatment, she looked ill and worn out, but she was very cheerful nevertheless. AGRIMONY was prescribed as her type remedy, because she bore the pain so cheerfully. IMPATIENS was given for tension. After three days she was able to report that she was much better although the stiffness remained in the shoulder. VERVAIN was added to the Remedies because she tried to use her left arm too much in her daily occupation in spite of the stiffness and the pain. Within another two days she reported that all of the stiffness was gone, and that she felt much better generally. The treatment was continued for several weeks until she could report that she was indeed fully cured.

Woman, age 63, unmarried. When she came to us for treatment, her entire body was affected by a skin irritation which at times caused her face to swell. She was normally a cheerful and healthy woman. Her house in London had been badly damaged by incendiary bombs during the war, and she had been treated for delayed shock at the time, but she had apparently recovered. Treatment was started in 1946. AGRIMONY was prescribed because of her cheerful disposition, and as her type Remedy. STAR OF BETHLEHEM was given because of the shock she had sustained, and HOLLY was added because it was observed that she hated the idea of having lost her home, and greatly resented the reason for it. After three weeks, she reported that the rash had nearly disappeared. She continued to take the medicine, and after one year she wrote again to say that she had been "entirely cured" although she did not specify the date, and that she was "entirely well again".

Man, age 42. He was a policeman, and he had a nervous breakdown following domestic troubles. He slept badly, and felt generally "unstrung" but he kept his troubles to himself, and he turned a brave face to the world. AGRIMONY, his type remedy, was given alone. After three weeks he reported that he was feeling fine once more, and that he was sleeping much better. He continued the treatment, and after another four weeks he said that he was much better, and that he no longer needed to take a laxative for constipation. Two months after starting the treatment, he wrote: "I now look back on my illness as sort of a nightmare. I am now fully recovered."

Baby, age 6 weeks, breastfed. The mother had been given penicillin for an abcess in her breast, and the baby developed a facial rash. The child was a happy little being. He slept well and did not seem to be restless or disturbed by the rash. AGRIMONY was prescribed as the type remedy, and CRAB APPLE was added to cleanse his body from the effects of the penicillin. Within two days the rash had disappeared, and the raised spots began to flake off. After one week, all of the symptoms of the rash had disappeared and never returned.

Extract from a letter received from a woman patient: "I am worried, and full of great fear as my gums are soft and spongy and I have not been able to wear my bottom dentures for four years. I was a normally happy woman, but this worry has got me down and I am afraid that my mouth will worsen and I shall not be able to eat anything." AGRIMONY was given for the worried state, and for the mental torture. ROCK ROSE was given for the great fear that amounted almost to terror. HORNBEAM was added to give her strength. After four weeks, she wrote again to say that her gums were beginning to harden; the same Remedies were repeated. Shortly thereafter, a setback occurred when she became resentful and impatient; her fears redoubled. The following Remedies were prescribed: AGRIMONY the basic Remedy, ROCK ROSE as before; WILLOW was added for her resentment, IMPATIENS for her impatience, and GENTIAN for the discouragement that the setback caused. After one month, she wrote to say that she was happier than she had been for a long time. She was feeling much better, and she could once again wear her dentures without any discomfort.

CHAPTER 3

ASPEN

Keywords: Vague fears of unknown origin; anxiety; apprehension

THE ASPEN fears are of the mind. They are the fears, the forebodings that come upon us for no known reason either by day or night. There might be a sudden awakening from sleep when terror sets in from no known cause, perhaps a bad dream which was forgotten; there might be the dread of going to sleep again lest the anxiety might recur. Often the ASPEN type fear is connected with thoughts of death or religion; it is the "goose-flesh" or the "hair-raising" fear of something not seen or heard; it is both sudden and unaccountable at the onset. It seems just to happen and the victim is assailed with a sense of disaster which is often followed by intense terror or emotional panic. It normally strikes when the person is alone, but sometimes the cold panic of inexplicable terror will swoop down when the person is among friends, when, humanly speaking, he should feel happy and safe. Those who experience this fear seldom speak of it to others, because since they can give no definite reason for their anxiety, they expect the misunderstanding of disbelief, and to be told that "it is all in the imagination". Dr. Bach wrote: "Fear of such things as an operation, a visit to the dentist, a thunderstorm, a fire or an accident are physical fears, and they are bad enough. But, they are nothing compared to an unknown mental fear which comes over you like a cloud, bringing fear, terror, anxiety and even panic without the least reason. These fears are often accompanied with trembling and sweating from the abject fear of something unknown. ASPEN is the Remedy for this kind of fear." The ASPEN fear is the exact opposite of the MIMULUS fear, for the latter is always from a known cause. The ASPEN fear is closely associated with the sheer terror of ROCK ROSE, for both often result in panic, emotional or physical.

Dr. Bach said of the positive aspects of ASPEN: "Fearlessness because of the knowledge that the universal power of love stands behind all. Once we come to that realization, we are beyond pain and suffering, beyond care or worry or fear; we are beyond everything except the joy of life, the joy of death, and the joy of our immortality. It makes the desire to invite experience, to invite adventure, knowing that it is leading us to our heavenly home and that we can walk that path through any danger, through any difficulty unafraid." There is an old Chinese proverb which says: "Fear knocked at the door; faith opened it, and there was no one there."

CASE HISTORIES

Woman, age 26, unmarried. She was of an extremely nervous disposition and was always frightened of something which she could not explain. When the fear came upon her she felt as if she was going to faint, and she very often did. She suffered from palpitations, and she felt that she lacked the courage to face life's problems. ASPEN was prescribed as the type Remedy for her inexplicable fear. LARCH was added to bolster up her confidence. After taking the medicine for a month, there was no appreciable difference, except that she had not fainted. At the end of the second month, she reported

that she had but one attack of fear, and that her heart palpitations had almost ceased. She said that she felt much
better in general. She continued the same treatment for
another two months, after which time she could say that "she
had never felt better physically" and that she was well able
to face any situation. She had lost her fears to such an extent
that her friends were asking her what treatment she had
taken that brought about such a noticeable improvement.

Woman, age 50. She had suffered since childhood from an
unreasonable fear that she might choke and suffocate. During
the last two years, this fear had so increased that she had
difficulty in swallowing, and she felt as if there were a tight
band around her throat. When she applied to us for treatment, she had been losing weight, and her vitality was at a
low ebb. An X-ray examination failed to reveal any physical
cause for her condition. She was given ASPEN as her type
Remedy, for fear without a foundation. She was instructed not
only to take it internally, in the usual manner, but also to
make a lotion of it, and to apply it to her throat three times a
day. The results were rapid and favorable. In three weeks
time she reported that she was able to swallow without discomfort, and that the unpleasant sensation of the tight band
around her throat had entirely disappeared. She was advised
to continue to use the medicine. Some few weeks later she
wrote to say: "I have completely forgotten that I ever worried
about choking."

Woman, age 60. Since childhood, she had been subject to
unreasonable fears which wakened her at night, and left her
in a state of fear and trembling, often with nausea, and a
dripping cold sweat. ASPEN was prescribed as her type
Remedy. STAR OF BETHELEHEM was added because of a shock
she had during her teen-age years. One month later, she
reported that she felt much better, but that she was suffering
from indigestion. Her sister had suggested that her symptoms
might be indicative of a cancer, and that terrified her. ROCK
ROSE was added to the Remedies prescribed before, to counteract the terror of a possible cancer. From that time on, her
progress was steady; her health improved greatly, and the

fears gradually subsided. Treatment was continued for three months longer, at which time she reported that all of her fears had vanished, and that she felt very happy again.

Man, age 60. He was a minister, and he had suffered a coronary thrombosis the year before. When he came to us for treatment, he said that he was filled with fear. He stated most definitely that it was not fear about his heart condition, but a fear from unknown causes, a fear without ground or reason. He had become very depressed and fatigued, and he had lost interest in his parish work. His voice was weak, and often failed him during his church services. He was given ASPEN as the type Remedy, for the groundless fears, and OLIVE for the exhaustion and its consequent depression. Treatment was continued for three months. At first he regained his strength as well as his interest in his parish work. At the end of the treatment, he reported that his voice was normal again, and that his old enthusiasm for his work had returned; most important, that he was no longer obsessed with unpleasant fears.

Man, age 80. For the past two years, he had an unreasonable fear of fire in his house. This caused him to become very nervous and irrational, for he would frequently dress himself during the night, and go downstairs to assure himself that all was well. ASPEN was obviously the type Remedy for a groundless fear. He was also given CRAB APPLE to cleanse the effect of his fear-filled mind, which had caused a chest congestion. After the first month, his wife wrote to say that he had improved greatly. He no longer went downstairs in the night, and the chest congestion was much better. He continued to take the Remedies for another two months when his wife reported that he was "altogether a different man, both mentally and physically."

CHAPTER 4

BEECH

Keywords: Intolerance; criticism; passing judgements

DR. BACH said about the BEECH type person: "It is obvious that none of us is in a position to judge or criticize, for the wisest of us sees and knows only the minutest fragment of the Great Scheme of all things, and we cannot judge, knowing so little, how the Great Plan will work." He also wrote: ["We need] to be more tolerant, lenient and understanding of the different way each individual and all things are working to their final perfection."* The BEECH type is an intolerant person who does not try to understand or to make allowances for the shortcomings of other people. Rather than trying to seek out the good qualities in others, the BEECH type tend to look for their faults, and to criticize them. The BEECH type persons generally lack humility, as well as the ability to put themselves in the position of the other fellow. They often fail to recognize the fact that the other person may not have had the advantages that they have had, nor the help of the experiences which they were privileged to encounter. Sometimes small habits, gestures and idiosyncracies of other people try them beyond measure; their annoyance is out of all proportion to whatever created their displeasure. This, indeed, is a true

---

* *The Twelve Healers and Other Remedies* by Edward Bach, The C. W. Daniel Company Ltd., Rochford, Essex, England; 12th edition 1969.

case of seeking first the beam within one's own eye. Here is a typical statement: "I have a strong and deep-rooted aversion to superficialities of all kinds; I demand and I seek exactness, order and discipline everywhere." This tendency toward criticism makes them rather lonely people, for they cut themselves off from the friendly, tolerant, companionship of their fellow human beings. The BEECH type differs from the WATER VIOLET person in that the latter are truly wise and understanding, and for that reason they may feel superior to those who are not treading the same path they are. It is this sense of superiority that brings forth a certain aloofness from the normal plodding mortal. Yet, the WATER VIOLET type never attempts to correct or to criticize those with whom he might disagree or even those to whom he feels superior.

Dr. Bach said of the positive aspects of the BEECH person: "[An example] of perfect tolerance. It was the Christ allowing the soldiers to place the crown of thorns on His head, to pierce His hands and feet with nails without His having one harsh thought. Instead He pleaded on their behalf, 'Father forgive them, for they know not what they do'."

CASE HISTORIES

Man, age 54. He was a bachelor who lived with his mother and his four sisters. As a person, he was always irritable and impatient, and could not tolerate his family's idiosyncrasies; to escape them, he tried to live in a dream world of his own making. He started to suffer from sciatica seven weeks before he applied to us for treatment. BEECH was prescribed as the type Remedy, for his intolerant attitude, and CLEMATIS for his attempt to escape into a dream world to avoid what he thought was unpleasantness. His first report was encouraging; he stated that he was free from the sciatic pain in the thigh, although the leg was still weak and, as he described it, "erratic". The same Remedies were repeated, and after two months he wrote to say: "The trouble in the leg has cleared up completely. I have decided to seek another job in a different town, and to live on my own. I shall then have a better opportunity to think of my family in a more understanding light."

Man, age 40. He was a commercial artist by profession. For over a year he had suffered from a rash on his face, arms, and hands. He was most critical of his physicians, and very irritated with them because they had failed to cure his condition. He was also critical of many things in general, or as he expressed it: "of humdrum things and humdrum people." He was becoming resigned to the rash, but it made him feel unclean. BEECH, his type Remedy, was prescribed for his critical attitude. CRAB APPLE was added as a cleanser for his skin condition. Sixteen days later, the rash had entirely disappeared, but he was fearful that it might return again. GENTIAN was added to the other two Remedies for his discouraged outlook. Nothing further was heard from him until two years later. He wrote to say that the skin condition had never returned, but that now he was suffering from a stiffness in both shoulders. BEECH, the type Remedy and CRAB APPLE were once again prescribed, because it was felt that a critical and rigid outlook remained. He wrote once more the next month to report that he was completely free of the pain and stiffness.

Woman, age 46. She wrote to us saying: "I am a reformer at heart. I like to change people, but I do not have enough humility to be a shining example. I am too intolerant. I suffer much pain due to toxins and inflammation caused by an incurable stomach obstruction." BEECH her type Remedy was prescribed for her intolerance; VERVAIN for her desire to convert all around her; CRAB APPLE because she ended her letter to us by saying: "I rather dislike myself." She took the Remedies for three months. During that period, there was at first but slight improvement, then suddenly she really became very much better. Her last report to us stated that she felt that she had become a different woman, and was now quite well.

Man, age 70. He was a most intolerant individual and critical of anyone who did not think as he did. He literally wore himself out saying: "Why does so-and-so think like that?" or "I can see nothing good in that man." He was irritable and cranky, and almost wholly without joy in his life. BEECH, obviously his type Remedy, was given alone. After some weeks, he was able to say: "I can see the fault in myself." He continued to take the Remedy and gradually he became filled with vitality and displayed quite an extraordinary sense of humor.

Woman, age 69. She was a thoroughly efficient person herself, but she was extremely critical of other people. She could not understand why they seemed unable to attend to details as she did. She did not, however, mention their faults to them directly, but she always felt very superior to them. In consequence of this attitude of superiority, she suffered from a chest congestion and bronchitis. BEECH was the type Remedy prescribed for her intolerance; CRAB APPLE as a cleanser, to remove the congestion in her chest as well as in her thoughts. She took these Remedies for quite a while before she acknowledged that indeed her outlook had changed greatly. She said that she had a much better understanding of the problems of other people, and of their difficulties. The congestion and the bronchitis had cleared up, and four years later she wrote to say that they never returned.

Man, age 52. He was retired, and he suffered greatly from an eczema of the scrotum, the skin of which had become dark and of a leathery texture. When he came to us for treatment, he had had the trouble for over two months. He was an intolerant and highly critical person, especially where the way-of-living of other persons was concerned. He was given BEECH, the type Remedy for his intolerant attitude toward his fellow men, and CRAB APPLE as a cleanser for his system. Within a month, the eczema had disappeared, and the skin of the affected area had become normal in texture. He continued to take the Remedies for another month. At that time he reported that his family said that they found him much more tolerant, and easier to live with.

Woman, age 55. She had suffered from liver and kidney trouble which she said had been greatly helped by a herbal therapy. However, a setback occurred, and she applied to us for treatment. She stated that she was a reformer at heart, and that she liked to change *others* whom she felt were on the wrong path. She wanted them to think the same way that she did, and when they did not comply, she became very intolerant of their lack of understanding. BEECH was the type Remedy, and she was also given CRAB APPLE to cleanse her thoughts as well as WHITE CHESTNUT because she said that she was unable to dismiss worrying thoughts from her mind. She reported some improvement after the first month, but as she said, she still lacked tolerance. The same Remedies were prescribed and after another two months she reported that her health had improved greatly, and that she had finally realized that she must let other people go their own way. She had learned that it was not her business to interfere in their lives, or to criticize them.

CHAPTER 5

CENTAURY

Keywords: Weak willed; too easily influenced; willing
servitors

THE CENTAURY people are quiet, sometimes timid,
lacking in individuality, docile and always willing to
do anything for others. They are submissive, easily
imposed upon and often become the prey of the un-
scrupulous people who take advantage of their good
nature. They are the "door-mats" that are both used
and overworked by others because they do not have
the strength of will to refuse; in this way they increase
the dominance of the bully. They become easily tired,
and often seem to be drained of their vitality. In
appearance they are often languid and pale, although
actually they are mentally alert, active, and wide
awake. In this they differ from the CLEMATIS people, for
the latter can be led and influenced because their
thoughts are elsewhere, and they have little interest in
the present circumstances. Unlike the HORNBEAM type,
the CENTAURY folk become tired because their vitality
is sapped by the over-doing of favors and responding
to requests from others, not because of any disinclination to do things. The CENTAURY type does not argue
or stand up for himself; he usually is quick to do the
bidding of others. His actions and thoughts are often
colored by the dictates and ideas of his companions
as well as by conventions. By not following their own
ideas or ambitions in life, they miss much of the joy.

independent adventure and experience can bring to them. Often they spend their lives unnecessarily bound to their family or their parents, and by doing this they neglect their own mission in life. They frequently enter their father's business instead of following an aptitude of their own, or they may wait hand and foot upon an ailing parent. In either case they ruin their lives by the servile attitude which chains them to an unsympathetic loyalty, even to the extent of foregoing marriage rather than leave the one who has enslaved them. Actually, they are servants, instead of willing helpers. CENTAURY gives strength to the mind and the body. It is most useful for weakness following a prolonged illness, when the patient feels too tired to make any effort on his own behalf, or when he is completely lacking in vitality.

The positive characteristics of the CENTAURY person is found in one who serves wisely, quietly, and unobtrusively. He knows when to give and when to withhold. Such a person is able to mix with his fellows and not lose his individuality; he is well able to support his own opinions and to follow the higher dictates of his inner self. He can complete his mission in life uninfluenced by the opinions of others.

CASE HISTORIES

Here is a letter from a typical CENTAURY person: "Mother has a terrific will power. I am sometimes almost afraid to offer any advice or suggestions. I dare not say how I long to go somewhere, even for a few hours on my own, as I would rather not go than face the inevitable upset. I am also feeling very tired, and while I long to get on with my painting, I find neither the time nor the energy. I would like to go to sleep; I feel so tired. I long to be able to plan things for myself. I long to get right away by myself and to rest and think and then do things when I am rested. A friend and his wife came the other day and insisted on taking me out. Mother was furious and said that they had no right to do so; they should have taken her too. How different from the attitude of my husband who simply said: 'How kind of them. I do hope that you enjoy yourself.' " CENTAURY was prescribed as the type Remedy, for her inability to assert herself, and she continued the treatment for three months. She gradually began to live her own life. She insisted that she have some time to herself each day to devote to her painting and to visit with her friends. Finally she gently but firmly insisted on going her own way, and much to her surprise, she found that not giving in to her mother's every whim, helped her mother greatly! Her mother began to become much more considerate of other people, probably for the first time in her life.

Woman, age 41. She was a mother of two children. She suffered greatly from insomnia, and she had practically not slept for the last twelve weeks preceding the interview. She had been given many kinds of treatments including electric shocks, but none had helped her much. When she came to us she had low blood pressure, she was anemic and felt exhausted, but worst of all she had lost interest in her appearance and in life in general. Her childhood had been a difficult one. Her father dominated the whole family and for him his children were simply slaves. She felt that she was a "nobody" and was continually working hard to gain approval. She was most sensitive to the opinions of others, and she felt a compulsion "always to do the right thing". CENTAURY the type Remedy was prescribed to free her from the domination of her father and from her slavish attitude toward conventions. HONEYSUCKLE was added to help her break from the bonds of the past, and OLIVE to strengthen the exhaustion of her mind and body. After the first month, her outlook was brighter. She wrote that she had taken up golf again, but that there was no improvement in her sleeping. ROCK WATER was added to the Remedies to help her relax and be less strict with herself so that she could enjoy the pleasures of life. The next month she said that she was sleeping better. Two months after that, her husband wrote to say that she now played golf twice a week, her interest in clothes had returned and she was enjoying life once more.

Boy, age 11. He was continually afflicted with bad colds and with influenza. This caused him to miss many days of school, and his education was suffering as a consequence. The family doctor had suggested a tonsilectomy. He was a rather self-effacing boy, and easily dominated by anyone with a will stronger than his. CENTAURY the type Remedy was prescribed together with HORNBEAM to give him strength; the continual colds had sapped his strength and vitality and even his desire to make any effort for himself. He took the Remedies for two months, and went throughout the winter without one cold; his health had improved so much that the idea of the ton-silectomy was abandoned. He also developed firm determination and a strong will of his own.

Woman, age 62. She lived with her aged mother, who was 91 years old. The mother had a very strong personality, and like a vampire, she sapped all of her daughter's energy until the daughter felt utterly exhausted in body and spirit. CEN-TAURY the type Remedy was prescribed to help her break from the domination of her mother. HORNBEAM was added to give her strength to cope with her daily duties. When she came to us she was also suffering from headaches and sinus trouble. After the first month she reported that she felt much better. Her headaches were less frequent, she felt less ex-hausted and she had much more energy. The same Remedies were repeated with the addition of HOLLY, because she wrote that she had some very disagreeable thoughts and emotions toward her mother. She was also advised to increase her social life and to go out with friends more frequently; in other words, to try to make a life of her own. Her final letter to us, after another two month period, indicated that she was well. The headaches and the sinus trouble were things of the past. She was able to control the disagreeable thoughts toward her mother, and she could finally stand up to her. She was also leading a life of her own, and she was an altogether happy person.

Woman, age 50. She was a cook by trade. She wrote to us: "My mother and sister are in a mental home. My father was very domineering, and made us do what he wanted all of the time. I still seem to be influenced by other people, and I do just what they tell me to do. I get so very tired that I cannot sleep and I cannot seem to stand up for myself." CENTAURY the type Remedy was prescribed. After taking two bottles of the medicine, she wrote again to say: "It is astonishing! I am so much better and I can even decide things for myself rather than do another's bidding."

Woman, age 67. She was married. She was of a very frail constitution, anemic, and was very much overworked at home. She had become anxious, depressed, miserable, and jealous because she was neglected. Although she did all that she could to help her family, she was under their domination, and could not stand up for her own rights. CENTAURY the type Remedy was prescribed to aid her in overcoming the domination of her family, and HOLLY because of the vexing thoughts her emotions generated. There was an immediate physical improvement; a bruise on her knee healed, and fibrositis in her back disappeared not to return, but the depression remained. The same Remedies were repeated over a period of four months, during which time she gradually improved physically and emotionally. Finally the depressions disappeared and did not return. She found that she was well able to stand up to her family and to assert her own rights. Laboratory tests established the fact that she was no longer anemic.

CHAPTER 6

CERATO

Keywords: Distrust of self; doubt of one's ability; foolishness

THERE are those persons who possess much wisdom, who are intuitive, who hold definite opinions of their own, yet they doubt their own ability. They are quite capable of doing foolish things by following the advice of others, against their own good judgement. Such is the CERATO type, and when they discover that the advice upon which they acted was unsound, they are apt to say: "I knew better. I knew that I should have done so-and-so." This is poor consolation indeed. A patient who sought the counsel of others wrote to us to say: "I found out that after having been advised by some friends to eat honey, it brought back all of my old symptoms. I should have known better, for honey has never agreed with me, and I have not eaten it for years for that reason." Sometimes, though rarely, the CERATO type will ask advice from others and then go their own way and use their own judgement. In illness, they are sure that a remedy will cure them until somebody tells them of a different one; they are inclined to try one medicine after another, always according to the latest recommendation. They are talkative people, for they are always asking questions, and in this way they tend to sap the vitality of others with their persistency. The CERATO type differs from the SCLERANTHUS person in that the latter cannot make up his mind between two choices, but he will eventually work out the decision for himself without asking the advice of others, unless of course it concerns a matter which calls for a qualified opinion. The CERATO person also differs from the CENTAURY type who is weak and thus easily persuaded, for the CERATO type does have a mind of his own, and contrary to the LARCH people, he has sufficient confidence in himself to stick by his decision once he has arrived at it. The CERATO folk have a great admiration for those persons who know their own minds, and who can reach a reasoned determination quickly. They even tend to imitate them so closely that at times it is possible to tell with whom they have been in contact, or what motion picture they have just seen!

The positive aspect of the CERATO type is quiet assurance. Such persons are very intuitive. They are sure of their ability to judge between right and wrong, and they trust themselves to act uninfluenced by any advice to the contrary.

CASE HISTORIES

Woman, age 68. She was a spinster and wrote: "I always know what I want to do, but I find that I must have it confirmed by the opinions of several other people, and when they don't all agree with me, I generally follow the majority vote, and mostly it does not end in the way I wanted it to. It is foolish of me I know, and people tell me that I tire them by asking so many questions. I get very tired too, and I suffer from sinusitis, very severely at times. I really feel desperate with the pain." CERATO was the type Remedy indicated because she could not trust her own judgement. CHERRY PLUM was added because of her feeling of despair about the pain of the sinusitis. After three months, the sinusitis had cleared up, and CHERRY PLUM was omitted from the next prescription. After taking the medicine for a total period of six months, she wrote to say: "I find that I don't have to ask others for their advice now. That is a great relief. I am also happy to say that I am no longer troubled with sinus pains."

Woman, age 55. She was a spinster who always had something the matter with her. It was either a cold, indigestion, a headache or a rheumatic pain; in any case she was seldom really well. Although she was quite capable of making decisions, she could not trust them. In the case of her health, this drove her from one form of treatment to another, and none was of much benefit. She was a talented woman who could do her work well and knew it. A person of many interests, she was continually making mistakes because instead of relying upon her own good judgement, she constantly sought the advice of others. When she came to us for treatment, she was very discouraged and depressed. CERATO the type Remedy was prescribed together with GENTIAN for her discouragement. She was treated for a long period of time. The physical complaints responded fairly rapidly to the Remedies, but it took a full two years before she was finally able to direct her own life, and to rely upon her own good judgement.

Woman, age 45. She was a nurse by profession, and had many years of experience. The hospital in which she had worked was about to be closed down, and she was to be transferred to the County Hospital. However, she had long had the desire to become a District Nurse, to visit patients in their own homes and in the nearby towns of the district. She had already taken and passed her automobile driver's test. Then, as she said, she suddenly lost faith in her own judgement. Though she wanted very much to be a District Nurse, she somehow felt that she should go to the big hospital. Confronted with this decision, she began to ask her friends for their advice. Fortunately for her, her friends (who would certainly appear to be both intelligent and true) withheld their advice, and were unanimous in suggesting that she make up her own mind, and that she do what she really wanted to do. CERATO the type Remedy was indicated and prescribed. She took the Remedy for about two weeks. At the end of that time she determined to become a District Nurse. She wrote to us to say: "Had my friends advised me to go to the hospital, I know that I would have been disappointed. I want to visit patients, and to work on my own."

Man, age 22. He was the son of a successful physician. When he came to us, he was approaching his final examinations in medicine. He was very unhappy, because he felt that he was not meant to be a doctor. He had always wanted to be an electrical engineer, but out of deference to his father's advice, which he had sought, he studied medicine. In doing so, he unfortunately went against his own inner conviction. CERATO the type Remedy was prescribed to give him confidence in his own decisions and IMPATIENS because he had become nervous and irritable. These Remedies helped him to see that he was not following his vocation in life, but he felt that he lacked the courage to make the necessary change. MIMULUS was added for the fear of making a change, and LARCH for his feelings of inferiority. He took the medicine for another two months. When he wrote to us again, it was to say that he had decided to give up further medical studies. He had gone to London "to take up the work I have always wanted to do". He was apparently very happy and had made many new friends. He said that he felt very well, and that at last he was making a success of his life.

Woman, age 72, a widow. She could never trust her own opinions, and was continually asking her friends what they would do if they were in her place, and what she should do about her poor health. The result was that she went from physician to physician, taking first one treatment, then another, always according to the advice she received, and generally without any benefit to her health. She had become very nervous about a large growth on her abdomen which she feared might be malignant, yet she was unwilling to have it removed surgically. CERATO her type Remedy was prescribed because of her inability to trust her own conclusions. ROCK ROSE was given for the terror that the thought of a malignancy caused, while HORNBEAM was added to give her strength. She took these Remedies for a period of three months. During that time the growth grew progressively smaller until it finally disappeared altogether. She became much stronger; her health was no longer a problem, and as she said: she resolved to put her foot down, and to make her own decisions.

Woman, age 33. She wrote to us saying: "I know what I really want to do, but I do not have sufficient trust in myself. I have followed the advice of my parents and of my friends most of my life, and I have never been happy or satisfied with my life or with my work. Now I have an urge to do what I want to do. Could the Remedies help me to be firm, and to follow this urge?" CERATO, the type Remedy was the only one prescribed. She took this medicine for six weeks, at which time she wrote again to say: "I have done it! Now, I feel that I can trust myself!

Woman, age 39. She wrote: "I married a good and kind man, but I never loved him. Now I feel that I must leave him, both for his sake as well as mine. I have met my real partner. My mind is made up, but I become filled with doubts and fears about my decision, and I ask advice from all and sundry. Their advice is usually contrary to my decision, but nevertheless I still keep on asking." CERATO her type Remedy was prescribed. She took the Remedy for three months. After that time she explained the situation to her husband who was a very understanding man. He granted her the divorce, and wished her happiness in her future life.

In the case histories cited above, CERATO enabled all of the persons concerned to arrive at a decision *by themselves*. Each developed the confidence to trust his or her decision, and each relied upon his or her judgement, regardless of what other people said or thought. P.M.C.

CHAPTER 7

CHERRY PLUM

Keywords: Desperation; fear of losing control of the mind; dread of doing some frightful thing

THIS Remedy is for the desperation and deep depression of those on the verge of a nervous breakdown. It is for those who in their despair contemplate turning to suicide as an escape. Here is a typical statement from a patient: "I lost my husband recently and ever since I have had a dreadful depression and a fear of the future. What is the worst of all, I have a terrible desire to end it all with an overdose." Another patient wrote to say: "I feel that I shall go out of my mind to the point of suicide." Such is the despairing and depressed attitude of persons who have undergone long continued mental torture or physical suffering. The distress becomes so great, that they fear the mind will give way under the strain. They fear that they will lose control of their thoughts or actions, and be impelled to do something dreadful or to commit an act which in happier times they would not consider for a moment. One wrote: ". . . I have an irresistible impulse at times to do my husband or my child an injury." There are also those who dread the thought of insanity, who fear that they might be going insane, as did the patient who wrote: ". . . a dreadful state of depression and a disturbed mind . . . I do not know how to go on, and I can no longer see my way out. It would be terrible to be shut up in an asylum." Yet again: "I have a feeling that I am going 'round the bend', that I am going 'up the wall'." And saddest and most dangerous of all, the patient who wrote and said that he had: "violent, almost murderous impulses which suddenly sweep across my mind. They result in my doing such things as pacing up and down, running, shadow-boxing mentally to settle an old score. I do not ordinarily feel like this."

The positive aspect is seen in the calm quiet courage and endurance of the prisoner of war for instance, who is undergoing mental and physical tortures, and who yet can retain his sanity.

CASE HISTORIES

Woman, elderly. She was recovering from a long illness and had invited a friend to come to stay with her. However, she found out that she could not get along with her. She then became very abusive toward her friend. She would strike out at her and shout hysterically. This was quite unlike her normal behaviour. Her friend left her, but this attitude continued toward all people with whom she came into contact and in fact became worse. CHERRY PLUM the type Remedy was prescribed for her lack of mental control. The result was remarkably quick, for she had but one more of these attacks. She was advised to continue to take the Remedy for another two months in order to consolidate her improvement.

Child, age 3½ years. The child was the twin of a much stronger brother, and indeed he had not been expected to live at birth, but he gradually grew stronger and survived. He had frequent screaming fits, and would throw himself on the floor, bang his head, and throw things about. He was constantly catching a cold, his appetite was poor, and he often vomited after eating. CHERRY PLUM the type Remedy, was prescribed to help him gain control over his feelings and SCLERANTHUS to steady down his variable moods. After four months, his mother reported that he had become a normal child. His general health improved, his appetite increased and the vomiting ended, and he was no longer subject to the screaming fits.

Man, middle age. He suffered greatly from sinusitis, and often had intense pain. He was a person who moved quickly, who was impatient and energetic, and these characteristics were aggravated by the pain from which he suffered during the attacks. He felt that he would go mad if he did not get some relief and that quickly. CHERRY PLUM was prescribed as the type Remedy for his desperate state of mind, together with IMPATIENS for his extreme mental tension. These were also prescribed as a hot fomentation for external application. To his great surprise, the very first night he had a fine sleep, and awoke to find the pain practically gone! He continued to use the drops and the fomentations for a few days more, and the condition was entirely cured. He has reported that after several years he has had no return of the attacks, but that he still takes the Remedies. He wrote: "I take the Remedies every now and then, for I have grown in patience, and I wish to continue in that condition."

Man, age 30. He came out of World War II suffering from shell-shock, and was very sensitive and high-strung. He had served through the entire war in the Air Force as a pilot, and the strain had just been too much for him. He had been given both drug and shock treatments, but neither of these had helped much. When he applied to us for treatment, he said that he was terrified that he might put an end to himself, and that he had an almost uncontrollable impulse to seize any knife or sharp instrument and "end it all". He slept little, and when he did, he had bad nightmares. He had lost his appetite, and was restless, thin and pale. CHERRY PLUM the type Remedy was prescribed for his desire to commit suicide. He took this medicine for a period of over two months. Gradually, during that time, he became less restless and the nightmares were not as frequent; he began to regain his appetite. ROCK ROSE was added to the basic Remedy for the effect of shock, and he took this combination for another two months. He continued to get better and better; although his progress was slow, it was certain, and he continued the treatment for a total period of about nine months. The Remedies were changed from time to time as his moods indicated the need for other combinations, but CHERRY PLUM, the type Remedy, was always included. At the end of the treatment, he was a different man, and he had regained his calmness and his confidence. He was able to return to his work; he ate and slept well, and had put on weight and looked very fit and healthy. He married, held a very responsible job and became a most successful business man. This happened almost twenty-three years ago, but there has never been even the slightest sign of a relapse.

Woman, age 42. As a child and as a young woman, she had always been a bright and cheerful person. She was separated from her husband who had been a cruel man. When she came to us for treatment, she told us that she felt as if life held nothing more for her, and that it was hardly worth while to continue the struggle to go on living. She was in a highly nervous condition and most excitable. She could not concentrate well. Her mind seemed to whirl about, and at times her body shook with involuntary tremors. She said that she only felt safe in bed; there she remained, thinking about suicide, and not going out of the house if she could avoid it. CHERRY PLUM was prescribed for the type Remedy, because of the loss of emotional control and the thoughts of suicide, and CLEMATIS was added because of her lack of concentration, and the fact that she lived in a dream world. Two months later, she was well enough to leave the house to visit with her friends. But the improvement was short-lived, and she felt once again that she was going to pieces, that she lacked energy, and that she was self-conscious. MIMULUS was added to the basic prescription as an antidote to her fear and nervousness, and HORNBEAM to give her strength of mind and body. She next reported that the medicine was doing her much good, and after taking it for another two months, she was able to write that she felt well again. She had found a good job, and she had regained her happy, cheerful outlook on life.

Woman, young, married. She had suffered from a nervous breakdown. Just before she was married, the chair on which she was about to sit was pulled from under her, as a joke, and she fell heavily to the ground. Ever since that accident, she wanted to hurt people, to scream, and to throw things about. She had an obsessive fear of one certain person, and she was terrified to go out of the house by herself, especially to do the shopping. When she came to us, she was very tense and depressed. CHERRY PLUM, the type Remedy was prescribed for her desire to hurt others, for her fear of committing a terrible act; ROCK ROSE for her terror of going out alone and WHITE CHESTNUT to calm her mind, and to help her gain control of her thoughts. Within one month, she reported feeling much more like her old self, and she found she was able to go to church alone. Within three months, she was able to concentrate on knitting, and even to enjoy it; she could laugh and smile because her fears were subsiding. Then she had a setback, and all of her fears returned once more. GORSE for hopelessness and discouragement was added to the basic Remedy of CHERRY PLUM. Progress toward better health resumed, and she was able to enjoy a happy Christmas with her family. She continued to take the medicine for a total of seven months, by which time she had completely recovered. Two years later she wrote to say that she had been happy and well, and that to her great joy, she now had a fine new baby.

CHAPTER 8

CHESTNUT BUD

Keywords: Failure to learn by experience; lack of observation in the lessons of life; hence the need of repetition

THIS is the Remedy for those people who tend to make the same mistakes over and over again. They do not seem to learn the lesson inherent in the experience. This may be because of indifference, or from hurry and inattention, or through lack of observation. Whatever the cause may be, they tend to create the same errors and to experience the same difficulties repeatedly. Finally, they may gain sufficient wisdom to learn how to deal successfully with such occurrences; only then will they be free of them. The CHESTNUT BUD type tries to forget the past, and there he is wholly unlike the HONEYSUCKLE person who tries so hard to remember it! This forgetting can be a good thing, but until the lessons of the past mistakes are understood, the CHEST-NUT BUD person has nothing to guide him for the future, and nothing to help him in the present.

The positive aspect of this Remedy is reflected by those persons who are keenly observant of all happenings, and especially of mistakes which occur. They tend to keep their attention in the present, and they gain knowledge and wisdom from every experience. They watch and learn from others. Dr. Bach wrote of CHESTNUT BUD: "This Remedy is to help us to take full advantage of our daily experiences, and to see ourselves, and our mistakes as others do."

CASE HISTORIES

Woman, age 20, unmarried. She was a college student. Every two or three months, she suffered from a very severe cold which would last a week or more in each case. In talking with her, it was discovered that she "welcomed" the cold, and that she found it a relief from the pressure of her work in college. She was filled with self-pity, and was completely unable to understand why these colds should come as regularly as clockwork. The first prescription was CLEMATIS because her interest was not really in her studies but rather in daydreaming, and CHICORY because of her self-pity. The colds were simply an escape from these conditions. That the Remedies helped was proven by the fact that her next cold was of only three days' duration. She was given CHESTNUT BUD, the type Remedy alone, after the ground had been prepared for it so to speak; she was very slow in realizing that her interest did not lie in her studies. Actually, she was wasting her time in the University, and she should have looked elsewhere to try to find congenial occupation. The results of the second prescription were excellent; she wrote to say: "I am leaving college for I realized that I must take up the work which I always wanted to do: domestic science. I have just become engaged to the perfect man. I feel wonderful, and I have had no more colds."

Woman, unmarried. She suffered from migraine headaches and bilious attacks ever since her childhood. She was a nurse by profession, and doing social work. She liked to escape and be by herself whenever possible; once alone, she became very sleepy, and lapsed into daydreams. She worried over many things; her work, as well as the health of her best friend. Though she blamed herself for all of her faults, she did not associate them with the migraine headaches. CLEMATIS was given as an antidote to her daydreams; AGRIMONY for her naturally worrying nature, which she did her best to hide; PINE because she blamed herself unreasonably. She reported in three weeks time; she felt better in herself and she worried less about her friend, but she had had two very severe migraine headaches. She had joined an art class, and she greatly enjoyed it, but she could not understand why she should have the headaches. The prescription was changed at this time to CHESTNUT BUD, the type Remedy, because she was so slow to learn that all of her life she had tried to escape from unpleasant realities into a dreamland of her own making. The next reports which we received were encouraging, and she finally wrote to say: "I have had no further attacks of migraine headaches nor of biliousness for the past three months. I feel much better, and much more alive. I realize that I had wanted to escape from my worries up to now, but now I can look them straight in the face, and confront them."

Woman, age 40, married. She had an ulcer on her right leg which would not heal. Though the ulcer was painful and prevented her from sleeping, she was of a placid nature, and never complained. Various combinations of the Bach Remedies had been prescribed for her, but the ulcer would heal only to break out again. She had become unhappy, discouraged and irritable. Finally CHESTNUT BUD was prescribed for her; it was felt that there was something in her nature that kept her from learning, and that was what caused the same condition to recur time and time again. GENTIAN was added for the discouragement and for the depression her failure to recover brought about. Her first report was encouraging. She had no pain for three weeks; the ulcer was definitely starting to heal, and she was sleeping better. The same Remedies were repeated twice more, and after a period of about four months, she reported that she was completely healed. One year later she wrote to say that there had been no recurrence.

Woman, age 76. For the past seven years, she had suffered from *tic douloureux* during the winter. The attacks were so painful that she could not touch her face without experiencing excruciating pain. She was in constant fear, day and night, that an attack would occur. When she came to us for treatment, she was discouraged and depressed. She herself said that she must have something to learn, but that she was apparently slow about learning it, because the attacks came every year! She was given CHESTNUT BUD the type Remedy, based upon her own remark about learning slowly; ROCK ROSE for her great fear of the attacks; GENTIAN for depression and discouragement. Three months later, she wrote to say: "I have felt exceptionally well thus far through the autumn, and I am hoping to go through the winter without an attack." She did not have an attack that winter, nor for that matter any other winter. Two years later she wrote again to say that the attacks had never recurred.

Woman, age 40, unmarried. She suffered from a periodic eczema in both ears and this made her feel unclean; she also suffered from headaches on one side of her head. She wrote: "I make the same mistakes again and again. I never seem to learn from experience, and each time that I make these mistakes, my ears break out with eczema." CHESTNUT BUD, the type Remedy was prescribed because she was so slow to learn and to profit from her mistakes; CRAB APPLE was added for the sense of uncleanliness brought about by the eczema. Her first report, one week later, indicated that her ears were clearing up. Two months later, the eczema had disappeared entirely, and she had no more headaches. Six months later she wrote again to say that all was now fine, and that there had been no recurrence of either the eczema or the headaches.

Man, middle age. He wrote to say that he had had an accident, and although he was suffering from a concussion, an *X*-ray showed no skull fracture. He was sent the RESCUE REMEDY immediately for shock and the concussion. He wrote again and said that his condition had improved within twenty-four hours and added: "I have had an acid stomach during various periods of my life and last year I suffered from an inflamed colon. This has recurred several times. I have responsibilities in my work, and I find that they are becoming a strain because I make the same mistakes repeatedly. In fact, when I look back upon it, I think that this may have something to do with my abdominal condition. All of my life I have been either slow of learning, or not observant enough, so I have had to do things over and over again." The Remedies prescribed were: CHESTNUT BUD, the type Remedy because of the need to repeat experiences; ELM for the strain of his work, and CRAB APPLE for his dislike of his physical condition, and as a mental cleanser. The improvement was gradual but seemed certain and then a setback occurred. GENTIAN was added to the original Remedies to combat this discouragement. Shortly thereafter, he wrote and reported that he felt well for the first time in his life. One year later, he wrote again to say that he had no further trouble, and that he was feeling better than ever before.

Girl, age 8. She was a child who was very slow to learn her lessons, and was always at the bottom of her class. Although she was not a daydreamer, and she was a bright and happy little girl, she was very careless about certain things. When she left home, she had to be reminded to take pencil and paper to school, and especially to look carefully before crossing a street. She was sometimes unaware of what was said to her; it was almost as if it did not register. She was also afflicted with a series of small boils. These caused her to be absent from school often and to miss classes. The Remedies prescribed were: CHESTNUT BUD, the type Remedy for her slowness to learn; CRAB APPLE to cleanse her system of any toxins. The first response was a physical one; the boils which she had in her ears disappeared, and never returned. The Remedies were taken over a long period. She gradually became more observant, and her memory improved. She did much better in school. Two years later, her mother wrote to say that she had been very well physically. She was happy and loved at school, and while she still did not stand too high in her class, her grades were at least passing, and the improvement was great in every way.

if a woman, usually bursts into tears at the ingratitude shown toward her. Another example from our files: "She becomes very cross when she does not get the attention she thinks is due her. She is given to a great amount of self-pity, and is apt to become tearful when she gets no sympathy. At the same time one is expected to do everything that she says." The CHICORY type person may even simulate or invoke an illness in order to keep friends and relatives waiting upon him and sympathizing with his unfortunate plight. It so often happens that children of domineering parents sacrifice their lives uselessly for such tyrants, unless they have the strength of character to break away from the octopus-like affection which binds them. They often forgo career or marriage to stay at home with such a parent, and in this way, they do not fulfil their own appointed mission in life; they become frustrated and unhappy indeed! The characteristics of the CHICORY type can occur in persons of all ages and of both sexes. An example of this kind of juvenile blackmail was found in a little boy who disliked going to school. As he lay in bed and demanded attention, he said: "I could *make* myself better if I could stay at home!" Another letter from a mother said: "My small son, age five, is starting school and I feel that I can't face the lonely future. I shall miss him so much, the house will be so quiet, it seems more than I can bear." This is an excellent example of purely selfish mother-love, and constitutes the outer end of the spectrum of selfishness. There was no thought that perhaps the child might be nervous or excited at school the first day; the only thought was that she might be distressed and lonely without him. The CHICORY persons give the appearance of doing everything possible for the happiness of others, while in reality they do so in a manner that brings neither peace nor rest to the unfortunate recipient of their selfish devotions for they only sap their vitality. They are the vampires of humanity who will stop at nothing to gain their own egocentric ends.

The positive aspects of the CHICORY type person is seen in one who is truly selfless in his care and concern for others; one who gives unceasingly, without the slightest thought of a return.

CASE HISTORIES

Child, age 6. She was a child who always wanted her own way and instigated arguments because they drew attention to her. She was a fussy child, critical and given to saying unkind things, yet at times, when her true nature showed itself, she could be most generous and cooperative. Her moods were subject to sudden changes. CHICORY the type Remedy was prescribed for her self-centeredness, together with SCLERANTHUS for her changeable moods. Her parents reported that good results were quite noticeable during the first few days. After a longer period, they wrote to say that the most remarkable changes had taken place in the child, and all were for the better.

Woman, middle age, widowed. Her only son was about to be married, and she suffered from extreme jealousy of her future daughter-in-law. Her attitude toward her son had always been most possessive, and now she was doing everything in her power to stop the marriage. She had developed various ailments; she said that she could not be left alone; she said that she would lose her house if he left her, and in any case her life would be finished. CHICORY was prescribed as the type Remedy for her egoism and possessive attitude, and HOLLY for her jealousy. After taking the Remedies for about two months, she did go to her son's wedding, and gave them her blessing. Nevertheless, it was a long while before she could forgive her son "for leaving her". She continued to take the Remedies for almost two years. She then wrote to say that she had made a new life for herself. She was now very fond of her daughter-in-law, and overjoyed with her grandchild.

Woman, age 61. She was a chronic worrier with a most negative outlook. She was critical of others, and always wanted to be the center of attention. She was house-proud, fussy about her garden and she could not stand being alone. For that reason she always tried to keep friends or relatives with her. When she applied to us for treatment, she was on the verge of a nervous breakdown, and she had a suspected duodenal ulcer. CHICORY the type Remedy was given for her self-centred attitude; WILLOW was given for her negative outlook and for her resentment of the happiness of others. After the first three weeks her family reported that she seemed to be much more cheerful. At the end of the first month, they wrote to say that "the improvement was marked and she was physically much better". After the second month they wrote again to say: "She has become quite a different person in her nature. She has also been very well physically, and the suspected ulcer did not develop."

Girl, age 9. Every Tuesday morning, she had such bad headaches that she had to remain home from school. When she was brought to us for treatment, it was discovered that Tuesday was the day when the assignment was a composition, and she was very bad at spelling. She disliked composition intensely, and the headache provided the excuse not to attend school on that day. The child was filled with self-pity. She was a little girl who wanted affection and attention, and she always tried to avoid unpleasantness, or doing anything which she did not like to do. CHICORY the type Remedy was prescribed for the self-pity and the need to be the center of attention. Her mother was advised to send her to school whether or not she had a headache. After two months, the trouble had completely disappeared, and she became a perfectly normal child. Now she is a fully mature young lady of twenty-five, and for the last fifteen years she has never reported having had another headache of that nature.

Woman, age 36. She was a professional singer. As a child she had been without love in her home, and she was greedy for affection and attention. She was filled with self-pity, and jealous to the extreme. When she came to see us, she was nearing total exhaustion. CHICORY was prescribed as the type Remedy for her self-pity and egoism; CHERRY PLUM because she had recently attempted suicide; HOLLY because she admittedly became ill with jealousy at the good fortune of her two sisters. The response to the medicine was excellent. After a period of six weeks she was able to say that she felt like another person, and that her concert performances had been better than ever before. As a result, she had signed a contract to sing in an opera, and wanted another bottle of the medicine "to see her through".

Child, age 6. She always craved attention, and had to have someone near her all the time. When she could not have her own way, she became fretful. When she was brought to us, she had had a sudden outbreak of a rash all over her body. The rash produced blisters, and she looked as if she had been burnt. CHICORY the type Remedy was prescribed for her fretfulness and self-pity, and CRAB APPLE as a Remedy to cleanse her system. After taking the medicine for a month, her grandmother wrote and said: "The little girl is quite well now. The rash has entirely disappeared, and she is much quieter and less fretful. She responded remarkably quickly, and now she is a happy little child."

CHAPTER 10

CLEMATIS

Keywords: Indifference; dreaminess; inattention; unconsciousness

Dr. Bach said that the following symptoms were common in varying degrees in the CLEMATIS types: a vacant,
faraway look; indifference; inattentiveness; preoccu-
pation; dreaminess; drowsiness; as a rule they are
heavy sleepers, and often they have a marked pallor.
The CLEMATIS folk *are* daydreamers and they *are* absent
minded. They live more in their thoughts than in their
actions. They lack concentration because their interest
in things of the present, and often in life itself, is but
half-hearted. They avoid difficulties or unpleasantness
by allowing their attention to wander, and by with-
drawing into a world of illusion and unreality. As one
patient remarked: "I withdraw into my own world, a
world of my own making, whenever there is something
unpleasant to face up to. I do it entirely automatically
now." Whenever they become ill, they make little or
no effort to get well, because they have so slight an
interest in life. It is almost as if they wish to leave this
earth, perhaps to join some loved one who is dead, or
just because life does not come up to their expectations
on this material plane. This lack of cooperation or
effort to get well Dr. Bach called "a polite form of
suicide". It was well named, because at times they
would rather die with a loved one than remain on
earth, and this is often the basis of suicide pacts. Un-

like the AGRIMONY temperament who seeks companionship to relieve his distress, the CLEMATIS person prefers to be alone with his thoughts. He is the opposite of the VERVAIN type, for he is listless, apathetic and inattentive, while the VERVAIN type is alert and full of interest. The CLEMATIS folk have poor memories, because with their thoughts far away, they seldom bother to listen or to remember what has been said. They may even pass a friend on the street without recognizing him when they are wrapped up in their own dreams. This lack of attention often affects the eyes and the ears, for those organs are being used for inward seeing and hearing only. For the same reason, the inattentive withdrawal may well be the cause of accidents on the street or on the highway. The CLEMATIS person needs much sleep; he enjoys dozing, and he can fall asleep almost anytime. Here is a typical statement: "I fall asleep while answering questions or while talking with a group of people. I almost invariably fall asleep when I attend church, or a lecture." The CLEMATIS type is mediumistic and sensitive to all kinds of influences for ill; he is impractical in everyday things. The CLEMATIS state may occur in any of us at any time when the mind is occupied with inner problems; joys or worries may also withdraw our attention from the present situation. CLEMATIS is the Remedy for fainting, coma, or for any form of unconsciousness, for all such conditions indicate a "loss of interest", whether enforced by circumstances or not, in present conditions.

The positive aspects of the CLEMATIS type is seen in those people who have a lively interest in all things, and minds that are sensitive to inspiration. Among these persons we find the practical idealist, the writer, the artist, the actor, the healer; in short, we find one who is master of his own thoughts, and who has great zest in daily living because he can fully appreciate the great purpose behind all of it.

Case Histories

Girl, age 12. The child had spots on her face. In spite of the doctor's assurance to her mother that they would eventually disappear, the child was greatly distressed, and lacked all confidence. She was a quiet, retiring child anyway, and always a daydreamer. CLEMATIS the type Remedy was prescribed for her general condition and her dreaminess. The child responded rapidly. She became much more lively, and interested in her school as well as in her home. According to her mother she became "almost eager" to do things. The spots faded away completely after the second bottle of medicine had been taken.

Man, age 37. He was sent to us by the firm which employed him, and in which he held an executive position of responsibility. During the last months, he had become indifferent toward his work, and seemed to be quite unconcerned over his failure to fulfil either his executive duties or his obligations to the firm. His wife had died the year before. He told us that he had always been a heavy sleeper, and had great difficulty waking up in the morning. He had been having difficulty concentrating on his work recently, but he seemed to be perfectly complacent about the whole thing and obviously he was not greatly interested in his daily affairs. His utter unconcern toward possible failure, his general lack of effort and his dreamy apathy indicated that CLEMATIS was the type Remedy. He took the medicine for two months. There was a steady improvement from the start, and the man was able to continue his work with an increasing efficiency. At the end of the two months, he had regained his normal state of capability.

—Extract from Dr. Bach's Case Records

Man, age 47. He had greatly overworked himself in the city for a number of years. During the last three months he suffered from an almost complete loss of memory. He was at times unable to remember his street address or his telephone number. He was sleepy during the day, and was indifferent toward his work. Seven years before, he had suffered a shattering domestic tragedy. His expression was vacant. He was completely apathetic and resigned to the fact that he had become useless. It was only with difficulty that his friends could persuade him to seek medical advice. For this apathy, the drowsy state and the absence of all interests, CLEMATIS, the type Remedy was prescribed. He took this for two months. Rapid improvement occurred, and he was able to resume his business and to work well. He was without the Remedy for one month, and there was a relapse. He resumed the medicine which he took for another two months, and since then the patient has remained well.

—Extract from Dr. Bach's Case Records

Man, age 38. He suffered from a temporary loss of interest in his work which was to rehabilitate maladjusted youths. He was by nature a keen and energetic young man, but he had qeen overworking, and when he came to see us he was sleepy, tired and depressed. His work had been badly affected, and he had received unfavourable reports from his superior. He hardly ever felt well and had catarrh in his throat which, as he said, "makes me feel unclean". CLEMATIS the type Remedy was prescribed for his loss of interest and for his sleepiness (which was only an escape from his work, which for the time being he disliked); CRAB APPLE for the feeling of uncleanness induced by the catarrh. He continued to take the Remedies for four months, at which time he was greatly improved. He had regained his eagerness and interest in his work and the catarrh had completely disappeared.

Woman, age 67. She was a typist. She said that all of her life she had been a daydreamer, even when she was working. In her leisure time she would doze off to sleep in her apartment, and awake to find that she had not done her housework. Loud noises or crying children disturbed her thoughts and tranquillity. All of her life she suffered greatly from chilblains on her hands and feet, even during the summer months. Since she tried to withdraw from the present conditions, it is not to be wondered that her circulation was poor! The withdrawal into a dreamworld caused a stagnation, both mental and physical. CLEMATIS the type Remedy was prescribed for her desire to withdraw from reality and to live in a world of her own making; CENTAURY was added to give her the strength needed to overcome the desire to escape from reality and the present. She started treatment in October. Though the weather was cold, she had only one bad chilblain on her big toe; otherwise, her hands and feet were not affected. She continued to take the Remedies, and in December she reported that she had some chilblains but that they were not nearly as bad as in former years, and that they were subsiding rapidly. She continued to take the medicine, and the next February she wrote to say that she could see great improvement in her hands and feet; she said: "I can work without gloves, a thing that I never dared to do before. My daydreams do not trouble me now." Two years later she wrote again to say: "I am remarkably well in every way. The chilblains have never returned."

CRAB APPLE

Keywords: The cleansing Remedy; despondency; despair

CRAB APPLE is the Remedy which cleanses the mind or
the body of that which it dislikes, and that which fills
it with despair and disgust. It is the Remedy which
restores to us our sense of proportion. There are times
when some negative quality in our natures may give
us a feeling of disgust or uncleanness. We may have
said something that was unkind, or have done some
cruel thing which was contrary to our true nature;
some habit which we are unable to break may make us
feel unclean mentally. CRAB APPLE helps us to see that
when a difficulty has been recognized, it is already well
on the way towards being totally eradicated. It might
also be that some physical condition such as eczema, a
rash, a blemish, a wart, a spot, a growth or a mole
might also make us feel unclean. These are the conditions for which CRAB APPLE should be prescribed. It is
the answer to the patient who wrote to us saying: "I
feel as if I want the same treatment that you give to
the radiator of your car when you find it stopped up
with rusty water." CRAB APPLE is also useful for over-
concentration of thought on some trivial matter, on
something that is of no real importance, but which
nevertheless occupies our minds and our thoughts to
the exclusion of things of much greater import. An
example is that of the mother who is more concerned
that the children wipe their muddy shoes before coming

into the house, than she is about their wet feet and the possibility of their catching cold. It is also for those persons who "have a bee in their bonnet"; for those who come for medical help, and report a spot on the face, but forget to mention a painful lumbago. Actually, these kind of people feel things so strongly that they become depressed and despondent with any treatment which does not quickly result in a cure. The Remedy is valuable for both internal and external use, for it can be used as a lotion, a compress or a hot fomentation. It can also be added to the normal bath; six drops of the prepared medicine is usually sufficient for the average-sized tub.

The positive aspect of CRAB APPLE is seen in those people who maintain complete control of their thoughts, and who have the wisdom to see things in their correct proportions. They are broadminded people who do not dwell upon trifles, and who realize that any manifestation of a physical disorder is due to an inner disharmony; thus it is within their own power to transmute it into harmony.

CASE HISTORIES

Woman, age 40. When she came to us, she had suffered for many months with a rash on her hands. Small hard lumps had appeared at the base of the fingers. The irritation was intense, and became worse when she felt nervous or tense. She was a kind woman, and normally a happy one. She was house-proud, and inclined to worry about trifles; things tended "to get on top of her" and she seldom found time to relax. The rash made her nervous about preparing the food for the family, and made her feel "unclean". CRAB APPLE the type Remedy was prescribed for her over-concentration on trivia, as well as for feeling of being unclean; VERVAIN was added to help her to relax and take things easy. Three weeks after starting the treatment, she reported that the rash and the irritation had ceased, and that the lumps were softening and starting to disappear. She added that for as long as she could remember she suffered from constipation; now, much to her surprise, the Remedies had given her complete relief from that trouble. She also said that she no longer worried about the house, and that was "a great relief, as I seem to have so much more time for other things". One month later she wrote again to say that her skin was now soft and healthy, the lumps had vanished, and she was no longer troubled with constipation. She said that she looked and felt at least twenty years younger.

Woman, age 65. Her work was to go to the homes of elderly people, to help them with the housework. She wrote: "Seeing so much distress, so much filth and dirt, has weighed on my mind, and I feel dirty too. I seem to concentrate on dust and dirt, and to look for it everywhere, even when there is no necessity to do so." CRAB APPLE the type Remedy was prescribed both orally, and as a lotion which she was told to put into her bath. Within two weeks, she wrote again to say that there had been a great improvement, and that now, quite often, she was able to shift her thoughts to happier things. She was not entirely cured, however. She continued to take the medicine for another two months when she wrote again to say: "It is wonderful to have clean and happy thoughts again."

Woman, age 70, married. By nature she was an active woman, and impatient with slowness in others, with noise, or with untidiness. When she applied to us, she was about to move into a new house. Her chief difficulty seemed to be a dislike of herself; she felt that there was much about herself that needed to be cleansed. She suffered from chronic bronchitis and a pain in the left side of the chest, as well as asthmatic breathlessness. CRAB APPLE the type Remedy was prescribed for the need she felt to be cleansed; IMPATIENS for her impatient and tense temperament. After the first month, she reported an improvement in the bronchitis, and a lessening of the chest pain. Next month she wrote again to say that there had been a definite improvement in her temperament. In spite of the annoyance of moving into a new house, she had remained quite calm about it, but she added that she felt tired. HORNBEAM was added to the original prescription to give her strength. Five months after the start of the first treatment, she wrote again to say that she was better in every way. The chest pains had lessened greatly; the breathlessness was a thing of the past, and she felt quiet and assured.

Boy, age 12. For the past year he had suffered from fits and fainting attacks. He had been working very hard at school to stand at the head of his class. Before the attacks started he had been well and happy, but now he suffered from frequent headaches, and had become very irritable. He had been fond of running, but since the first attack occurred during a cross-country run, he had been forced to give up that sport. He had a very violent reaction to the drugs which were given to him; the attacks increased, he had double vision, and he started to lose the use of his right arm. It was then discovered that he suffered from infected tonsils which the doctors felt were responsible for his frequent head colds. The tonsils were removed; his general health improved slightly, but the fainting fits continued. He was given more medication with the result that the attacks recommenced and he lost his memory. The medication was changed again, and this time the drugs affected his speech, and caused him to fall into a deep sleep. He was getting more worried and more irritable, so medication was finally suspended, and he felt better without it. Then it was that his parents sought the help of the Bach Remedies, and he was brought to consult with us. It was our opinion that the first step should be clear to his system of the toxic effects of the medication which he had been given. To this end, CRAB APPLE was prescribed as the cleansing agent; CLEMATIS was added for the loss of memory and the "escape from the present" that occurred during the attacks; ROCK ROSE was added to combat his fear of the fits returning. After taking the Remedies for one month, he wrote to his mother from his school that he was getting much better, and his mother added in her letter to us that the whole tone of his letter was much more alive. Two months later she reported to say: "He is very much better, and working for his college entrance examinations, but he is worried about his loss of memory. He has had no more attacks." WHITE CHEST-NUT was added to the basic prescription to help him over-come any worry either about the possible loss of memory, or forthcoming examinations. One month later his mother wrote again and said: "His headmaster describes the result as a miracle. He has made a remarkable recovery, and he has even been doing cross-country runs again with no ill effects at all. He is practically normal now." The Remedies were continued for another two months, and since that time there has been no recurrence of any trouble.

Woman, age 63. She had separated from her husband a few years before, and she was still very resentful toward him. Though she had had two operations, and was under constant medical supervision, a chronic uterine discharge persisted, and this gave her a feeling of self-disgust. When she came to consult with us, she was impatient and irritable. CRAB APPLE was prescribed for her feeling of self-disgust; WILLOW for her continuing resentment toward her husband; IMPATIENS for her irritability. Her first reaction to the Remedies was an emotional one; she became decidedly less irritated, and despite the fact that the discharge persisted, she accepted the fact more philosophically. She continued to take the Reme-dies for six months, at which time she wrote to say: "I am cured of the discharge after thirty years! I am more con-tented, I keep myself busy and active, and I have many interests in life."

Woman, age 43, single. Outwardly she appeared to be a cheerful and friendly woman, but she concealed her true sentiments from others. Inwardly, she held feelings of self-loathing because of a bad psoriasis on her face, neck and ears. She had this condition for many years, and no treatment had helped it. Recently she had been told at the place where she worked "not to show her face there again". This cutting remark was a cruel shock to her. The Remedies prescribed were: CRAB APPLE because of the feeling of uncleanliness; AGRIMONY, her type Remedy, because she was of a friendly, cheerful disposition; STAR OF BETHLEHEM for the shock she had received. She was also advised to bathe her face with milk in which some drops of the medicine had been mixed. After two weeks she wrote: "The results are wonderful in every way. The skin is not so irritated and the flaking is less. The milk lotion has worked wonders. I am going back to work again, and I am much calmer now." The Remedies were continued for another three months, during which time she suffered one setback which was due to worry and stress because she became depressed and discouraged. GENTIAN was added to the basic prescription for the discouragement. Improvement was certain and rapid after that. She finally wrote to us to say: "It has been a very long time since I felt so well or since my skin has looked so well. You can realize how confident I am now when I tell you that I am going to the United States to work."

CHAPTER 12

ELM

Keywords: Occasional feelings of inadequacy; despondency;
exhaustion from over-striving for perfection

THIS Remedy, which is made from the flowers of the
Elm tree, is for those who at times feel overwhelmed
by the responsibilities and scope of their work. There
are times when one feels that the results of his efforts
are inadequate, and this brings about a state of
despondency and exhaustion. The ELM type persons
are very capable, efficient, and intuitive. They often
hold positions of importance. They may be key men in
industry, Ministers of State, physicians, teachers,
nurses. In every case they invariably have others dependent upon their decisions, whether it concerns
matters of State, or being the head of the family. All
of those persons who hold positions of trust because of
their ability, their wisdom, or their soundness fall into
this class. Decisions of importance depend upon their
advice, and they may even be the only persons suited
to certain jobs; they come near to being indispensible
in whatever capacity they serve. The ELM folk know
that they have capability to do all that is required of
them, and to do it well. They have chosen their work
in life, and they are well aware that it is their mission.
Yet there may be occasions when the very magnitude
of the responsibility causes them to feel that it is
humanly impossible for one person to assume it. At
this crucial moment they could feel that they are not

equal to the job. This is the moment when they might fail, and in failing, bring about a catastrophic condition which could result in untold distress and hardship to others. Any momentary doubt of their own abilities leaves them feeling weak and exhausted. Fortunately, this feeling of despondency does not last long. They are quick to recover their stability because of their inner conviction that they have been chosen for this particular type of work, and they will always be given strength and wisdom to achieve the task. The ELM exhaustion differs greatly from the two other types, HORNBEAM and OLIVE. The HORNBEAM person suffers fatigue through a dislike for the work he is doing, while the OLIVE type is worn out by long and continued suffering or stress. Always bear in mind that the ELM exhaustion is *temporary*; it is a momentary faltering of self-confidence, but, during this brief moment judgement can be dulled, wisdom overclouded and experience forgotten.

The positive aspects of the ELM character are manifest most of the time; outstanding among them are self-assurance and confidence. These virtues are the result of an unshakable inner conviction that help will always be forthcoming when needed. It is another praiseworthy aspect of the ELM folk's character that their powerful abilities are generally directed toward the safety, the welfare or the betterment of others.

Case Histories

Man, middle age. He was a clergyman. For some time he had suffered from bronchial trouble, and he had lost confidence in his ability to resume the trying duties of a large parish. He felt that he was inadequate, and he had become very depressed. ELM the type Remedy, taken alone for a month restored him to his usual cheerful self, and gave him the confidence and strength to resume all of his normal duties.

Woman, age 45. When she applied to us for treatment, she was suffering from acute nervous tension and was taking drugs for insomnia. She held a responsible job, and had a large staff under her. The pressure of the work had been heavy. Although she knew that she could cope with it, she was beginning to feel that perhaps it was too much for her. This thought depressed and exhausted her. ELM the type Remedy was given to counteract the belief that her tasks were beyond her strength; WATER VIOLET because she was naturally a quiet, efficient and capable person. After two weeks she reported: "The effect was immediate. The nervous tension lessened at once and in a few days it disappeared. I stopped taking any drugs for insomnia and after the first few nights I have slept normally. I am now well, and once again I know what the joy of living is."

Woman, age 38, married. She was the mother of five children, and was left to care for them after the sudden death of her husband. Although she was a very capable housewife and mother, she told us that she felt that she could not look after her children and educate them; she felt the responsibility was too great, and she was in a very deep state of depression. She was given ELM the type Remedy, to fortify her with the knowledge that she would be helped to do all that was necessary, and STAR OF BETHLEHEM for the shock of her husband's death. She took the medicine for two months. By that time she was able to resolve her problems efficiently, and the depression had left her. As she said, she had no time to think about herself.

Man, age 65. He was a very successful Bach practitioner, and was busy all day long treating patients. He suddenly felt overwhelmed by his work; he felt that he could no longer cope with all that he had to do. This brought on a state of exhaustion, and depressed him greatly, because he loved his work. ELM the type Remedy was prescribed for the temporary state of mind occasioned by the belief that he could no longer do his work. One bottle of the Remedy restored him completely within two weeks.

Woman, age 50, unmarried. She was a very capable and efficient woman who held a position of responsibility. Since her childhood, she had always suffered from insomnia. She had consulted with many physicians over the years, but without results. When she came to see us, she was always tired, and felt as if she could not go through her day's work. ELM the type Remedy was prescribed for her confidence and ability; HORNBEAM to give her strength to do her daily work. Within a short period she was able to write: "The Remedies worked almost immediately and I felt greatly relaxed for the first time in years. After the first week I was able to sleep the night through without taking any pills, and I feel that I do not need them any more. I could hardly dare believe what had happened. Now that I am well, I know what happiness means! It is almost too good to believe!"

Woman, young, married. She had three children, and wanted more, but she was suffering from extreme exhaustion which no treatment that she had undertaken could help. She felt heavy upon awakening, and all day long she was sleepy and unrefreshed. She was a person with a great sense of responsibility, and she became very worried that she would be unable to look after her family as she felt she should. ELM the type Remedy was given for her great sense of responsibility; OLIVE for her exhaustion. Within six weeks she had recovered and was able to write: "I have never felt so well in my life before." The next year she wrote again to inform us that she had given birth to a baby boy.

Man, middle age. He was a highly sensitive and dynamic person. He was working at a high creative level, and demands were heavy upon him. He had acute attacks of bronchitis, and when he applied to us, he was suffering from utter exhaustion. ELM was the type Remedy prescribed, so that he might be able to continue the exceptional work to which he was dedicated, work which threatened to devitalize and overwhelm him at times; OLIVE was added for mental and physical exhaustion; VERVAIN for his enthusiastic and active mind. He took this medicine for quite a long time. Eventually his health was so improved that he could carry on with his exacting work according to his own high standards.

Woman, age 50. She was the headmistress of a school, a position of heavy responsibilities. She wrote to us saying: "I can cope with the larger things of life better than with the smaller. I was called upon to assume heavy obligations at an early age, but now, at times, the responsibilities of the school seem to overwhelm me." She was a most conscientious and thorough person in her work. She suffered from varicose veins, a condition made worse by the long hours of standing her work required. ELM the type Remedy was prescribed because she felt that her task was beginning to overwhelm her; HORNBEAM was added to give her strength for her daily work. After taking the medicine for four weeks, she wrote: "My changed outlook is unbelievable. I never thought it possible to regain the clear untarnished thoughts of my earlier years! The veins in my legs do not ache as much as they did before." She continued to take the Remedies for some time longer. She then changed to another school where she was not required to stand so much, and where she had more opportunity to rest. Although the varicose veins never entirely disappeared, the pain went and never returned again.

CHAPTER 13

GENTIAN

Keywords: Doubt; depression; discouragement

GENTIAN is the Remedy for those whose outlook is negative and who suffer from deep depressions and dark melancholia. It has been said of the GENTIAN type that "He wouldn't be happy if he was happy". The GENTIAN folk are easily discouraged when things go wrong or when they are faced with difficulties. They falter and become despondent at setbacks, whether from an illness or from the affairs of daily living. They refuse to believe that it is their own lack of faith and understanding which prevents them from overcoming difficulties they believe to be insurmountable. They fail to understand that their own negative state of mind attracts those very conditions. The depression a GENTIAN person experiences is always from a known cause. Thus it differs from the intense gloom of MUSTARD which descends upon a person with no apparent reason. GENTIAN is a valuable Remedy to use in any illness where there has been a setback that discouraged the patient. It is also useful for children who have become discouraged by their examinations or schoolwork.

The positive side of the GENTIAN nature is fine indeed. Such people understand that there is no failure when one is doing his utmost, whatever the apparent results may be. They know that there is no obstacle too great, nor any task too big to be undertaken with the conviction that it can be accomplished.

CASE HISTORIES

Woman, age 50. Following a hysterectomy, she felt over-tired and suffered from acute attacks of depression whenever anything went wrong. She said that she "felt like a fool to be so discouraged". GENTIAN was prescribed for the depression, and OLIVE for the weariness. Within a month, she reported that she had no more attacks of depression, and that she felt better in every way.

Man, age 39. He had suffered from asthma since babyhood and throughout his entire life. He had tried many forms of treatment, and now, when he came to us, he was very dis-couraged, and was resigned to life-long suffering. When the attacks were severe, they lasted about three days. He worried, secretly, that he might lose his job through the ill-ness; he was a widower with one small son. Although, as he said, he had strong doubts that the Remedies could help him, he nevertheless decided to give them a try. The Remedies prescribed were: GENTIAN the type Remedy for his pessimis-tic and negative outlook; AGRIMONY for his efforts to hide his worries about his condition; WILD ROSE for resignation to his condition. He took the Remedies for three months. To his surprise and delight, he suffered only one severe attack during the time, and that was at the start of the treatment; he still had occasional difficulty breathing at night, but he was sleeping much better. At the end of another three month period, six months from the time that he started the treat-ment all asthmatic attacks had stopped, and never recur-red. He was in good health, and sleeping normally again.

Man, age 40. Following a nervous breakdown five years before, he had periods of extreme nervous tension, and attacks of depression. He became easily discouraged, and expected things to go wrong. He felt very nervous and that "everything depended on him". GENTIAN was prescribed for the depression and the discouragment; MIMULUS for the nervousness and anxiety. At the end of two months, he reported that his life was now much brighter, and that he was able to deal with his problems.

Woman, age 51, married. She had been a patient in a psychiatric hospital suffering from melancholia. Her husband wrote to us and said that since her release she had improved, but she still suffered from depressions and anxiety. He went on to say that she was very weak, without an appetite, and that she slept badly. GENTIAN was prescribed for the depression and melancholia; ROCK ROSE for her fears; HORNBEAM for her low vitality. After one month, the husband wrote again to say that she had made very good progress; physically she was much stronger, and was able to her housework. He also reported that though she was not able to concentrate fully, her memory had greatly improved, her depressions were less and her appetite had returned. After another month, he wrote to say: "She is her old, cheerful self once more."

Man, age 72, a retired army Major. He had had Ménière's disease fourteen years before he wrote to us, but he had a spontaneous remission, and the effects disappeared by themselves. Now, the disease had returned; he wrote: "I find my life miserable. I am unable to risk going anywhere. Between attacks, I believe that the disease has gone for good, but when they return, I am down in the depths again. I have become very fearful of these attacks." GENTIAN was prescribed for his despondency; ASPEN for his apprehensiveness; SCLERANTHUS for his indecision, which, incidentally, was quite foreign to his natural character. After a month, he was much brighter in spirit, and he looked much better. He had one or two threatened attacks, but they had not developed. Shortly thereafter he wrote again to say that both the attacks as well as the dizziness had definitely ceased. He said that he felt and looked better, and was able to go out without fear of an attack. Finally, he said, he was once again able to make decisions.

Man, age 62, a dental surgeon. He had digestive troubles for over a year, with abdominal spasms, flatulence and diarrhea. In spite of the assurance of his physician that his condition was not serious, he could not bring himself to believe it. He became depressed, worried and fearful. He lost weight through constant worry, and imagined the worst.

When he felt well, he was buoyant, but when he was depressed, felt that he was going to die. He had no pain after eating, only much gas; he slept well in spite of everything. GENTIAN was prescribed for his depression and doubt; SCLERANTHUS for the alternating moods which swung from elation to depression. The first report received from him indicated that he felt very much better and that he was recovering some of his composure. The next report stated that the flatulence had greatly decreased, and that emotionally he felt much more stable. His final letter indicated that he was very well; there was no pain, no flatulence, and most important, no anxiety about his health. He had returned to normal, physically and emotionally.

Woman, middle age. She had become disheartened on account of poor health. She suffered from poor circulation, constipation, and she had a whitlow on the middle finger of her left hand. There would be times when she would feel slightly better, but then she would relapse and become discouraged again. Her outlook on life was gloomy, and her thoughts were negative and depressed. GENTIAN was prescribed for her depression and discouragement; WHITE CHESTNUT for the negative and unpleasant thoughts which continually circulated in her mind; CRAB APPLE as a cleanser of mind and body. The whitlow soon cleared up, and the constipation became much better. She continued to take the Remedies for three months. When she visited us at that time, she declared that she felt much better in herself. The constipation was no longer a problem, and she was beginning to feel that life was worth living once again.

Woman, age 70, married. She lived with a sister-in-law with whom she was wholly incompatible. By nature she was a cheerful and contented person, but she became easily upset and discouraged when anything went wrong. When we first saw her, she had literally given up; she had lost interest in life and lacked the strength to make an effort on her own behalf. She pictured herself as an invalid, and it was with difficulty that she could get up from a chair, or climb the stairs. GENTIAN was prescribed for her depression and discouragement; WILD ROSE for her lack of interest in life; HORNBEAM to give her strength. Four weeks later she was able to walk about the house and to climb the stairs alone. After that she had improved still more, in body and mind, to the joy of everybody near her. She had established a friendly relationship with her sister-in-law, and she was again able to do her full share of the housework.

CHAPTER 14

GORSE

Keywords: Hopelessness; despair

GORSE is for those who have lost heart and suffer from hopelessness and despair after the failure of many treatments to help them. It is for those who have been told that there is nothing more that can be done and who therefore feel that they must continue to bear their pain and suffering for the rest of their lives. It is for the person who feels that it is useless to try further treatment, but just to please a relative or friend they will "try once more", although, as one patient said: "I know that it will do no good." The Remedy is also of value in illness of long duration, especially in those cases where progress has ceased after some improvement. GORSE is also very useful to give early in any chronic case; it will give the patient a hope of recovery, and that is the first step towards a cure. It should also be used where the patient is convinced that some inherited condition, or tendency, has condemned him to a lifetime of suffering. Dr. Bach said of the GORSE type: "They are generally sallow, and rather dark of complexion, often with dark lines beneath their eyes. They look as if they needed sunshine in their lives to drive the clouds away."

The positive aspect is found in those persons who have a positive faith and hope, and a certainty that in the end they can overcome all difficulties. They are not influenced by their present mental and physical condition, nor by the advice or opinions of others.

CASE HISTORIES

Woman, age 52, married. During her interview, she said that all during her life she had been inclined to look upon the dark side of things. Now she was feeling utterly hopeless; she had given up trying or even hoping to regain her health. As a result of this negative outlook, she had suffered for years from bronchitis and colds. At night, she had the feeling of suffocation and a chronic cough; she could not sleep well, and she generally awoke with a headache in the morning. She had tried every cure that she had heard of without success, and she frankly stated that she had little confidence that the Remedies could help her. GORSE the type Remedy was prescribed for her hopelessness; HORNBEAM to help her to regain the strength to cope with life again. Her first report was encouraging; she stated that she felt brighter and less depressed, and that she saw a ray of hope. Her cough had improved, and she felt less fatigued. The same Remedies were given for the next two months. This time she wrote to say that she was much more optimistic; the feeling of suffocation had disappeared, and she was no longer fatigued. Furthermore, for the first time in years, she was sleeping well. The cough remained, but she felt that it was occurring at less frequent intervals. VERVAIN was added to the original Remedies to reduce a tension and sense of strain occasioned by her having to do her own housework, whether or not she felt up to doing it. She took these Remedies for another two months, when she wrote again to say: "I feel a different person altogether since I have been taking the Remedies." She went to Canada, and continued the treatment for another five months. She wrote once more to say that she felt fine, and that the cough had finally disappeared and none of the former symptoms had returned.

Man, age 51. For the last twenty-eight years, he had suffered from psoriasis on his legs, with irritation and scaling. This affliction, which had been brought about by a period of anxiety and worry, caused him great mental torture and despair of ever being cured. He was inclined to be over-serious by nature; although he did have a sense of humor, he could not suppress a feeling of disgust engendered by the disease. He was frankly hopeless of being cured, but to please his wife he agreed to consult with us. GORSE was prescribed for the extreme hopelessness and the long duration and stub-bornness of the ailment; AGRIMONY to combat the mental torture the psoriasis caused him; CRAB APPLE for the self-disgust and as a cleanser of mind and body. Four weeks later, he wrote and said: "I feel better in myself, and more hopeful. My skin is less irritated than it has been for a long time and the amount of scaling is negligible, while the sores are decreasing in size." Treatment was continued for six months, after which time he was able to write: "I have never felt so well in my life. It is almost impossible to believe that I have been cured of my long-standing condition. I am getting better each day."

Man, middle age. He was a true pessimist who had never expected much from life, and who was continually depressed. Ten years before he consulted us, when he was in the Navy, he suffered from deeply cracked hands in the winter, and scaly skin in the summer. These conditions had persisted since that time, and he was quite despairing and hopeless that a cure could be effected. GORSE the type Remedy was prescribed for his hopelessness; CRAB APPLE to cleanse his mind and body. He reported that for the first two days he was sleepy and listless, but that after that he began to feel more active, gaining vitality. The hands began to heal, but when the weather turned colder he suffered a setback which discouraged him. The treatment was continued for another month when he reported that he had "a feeling of general fitness, a much more lively mind, and a total healing of my hands." The treatment was continued for another two months. None of the symptoms have returned.

Man, middle age. He said to us that he had never really felt well in his life. He suffered from numerous minor ailments and from severe headaches which annoyed him greatly. He had tried all kinds of treatments, but nothing seemed to help. He said that he was only trying the Bach Remedies to please his friends, that he himself had little faith that he could be cured. GORSE the type Remedy was prescribed for his hopelessness; IMPATIENS was added to counter his irritability and annoyance. At first his progress was slow; after some weeks, he said that the headaches, which he had all of his life, were gone. In the following two months he made slow progress but after that he wrote: "I have gained a sense of humor and I get a lot of pleasure out of life because I feel so well."

Man, age 50. For years he had an agonizing pain and swelling in his left hand which was almost unbearable, and at times incapacitated him. He had become depressed and hopeless after trying many treatments without any success. At the urging of a friend, who had benefited from the Bach Remedies, he consented to try them. He wrote saying: "I cannot get any sleep at night which makes me very depressed at times." GORSE the type Remedy was prescribed for his hopelessness, and because of the long duration of the complaint. He was instructed to use the Remedy both orally and as a lotion to bathe his hand with. He wrote again, after one month, to say that he was feeling better; he could sleep again, and the swelling on his hand was becoming less. He continued the treatment, and after another two months he was able to report: "I am feeling quite well now, thanks to your treatment. All swelling and pain in my hand has gone." The treatment was continued for another month, but the symptoms never returned.

Man, age 59. He contracted a serious double pneumonia for which he was given penicillin. The doctor held out little hope for his survival. During the crisis, his wife gave him repeated doses of the RESCUE REMEDY* and he pulled through the crisis and lived. When he called upon us for treatment, he was in a very weak condition; his heart had been strained, and his breath came in short gasps. He was coughing blood,

---

* For description of the RESCUE REMEDY and CASE HISTORIES, see Chapter 40.

and he felt hopeless and despairing. GORSE was prescribed for the despair and hopelessness; OLIVE to give him courage and strength after his grave illness. Within a few days he was able to sit up for an hour at a time, and he increased the time every day. His whole attitude had changed. He said that he knew, now, that he would get well. He gained strength daily, and the blood in the sputum was almost absent. He continued the treatment for four months, at which time he had completely recovered.

Man, age 63. For as long as he could remember, he had always had a slight sinus trouble, but it had become increasingly worse during the last eighteen months. About nine months before he applied to us for treatment, he had developed a thrombosis in his left leg, and he had to be hospitalized for some months. When he called us for treatment, he was at home in bed because he could not walk. He said that since his retirement, he had just gone to pieces. Now he was hopeless, filled with despair, and fatigued. GORSE the type Remedy was given for his great hopelessness and despair. Within three weeks, he reported that he was certainly feeling better; he was sleeping well, and his appetite had returned. GENTIAN was added to the original Remedy to give him further encouragement, and in another month he reported feeling wonderfully well. He was walking, although his knee was stiff, and he had to have physical therapy for this condition. Three months later, he was very well and felt an entirely different person. He was anxious to resume his activities, and his hopelessness was a thing of the past. His sinus no longer bothered him, and his knee was perfectly well.

Note: In every case, it will be observed that when the patient began to feel brighter and happier, more hopeful and less depressed, the body responded quickly, and the cure was assured. P.M.C.

CHAPTER 15

HEATHER

Keywords: Self-centeredness; self-concern

HEATHER people are always concerned about themselves. They are filled with their ailments, their problems, and even the trivia of their day. They like to tell others about their difficulties, and to discuss them whenever they can. The HEATHER type talks rapidly and incessantly, always bringing the topic of conversation to themselves. Here is a typical remark about a HEATHER person: "She must always be the center of interest. At table, she always tries to steer the conversation back to herself or to her house. Her grandchildren make bets on how quickly she can turn the conversation to herself!" Another wrote: "She talks to all and sundry about her trials and tribulations." The HEATHER people like to come close to you, to speak into your face, and for this reason Dr. Bach called them "buttonholers". Their excessive self-centeredness saps the strength and vitality of their listeners, leaving them completely exhausted. For this reason, they are often shunned and avoided. It is difficult for their companions to escape from them, for they try to hinder their departure. Since they take the vitality of others and live on it, they dislike being alone and they become unhappy when they are by themselves. They fear solitude for this reason. They do not suffer from self-pity; rather they enjoy making mountains out of molehills. They are poor listeners, and have little interest in the problems of other persons. They are the exact opposite of the AGRIMONY type, who always try to conceal their problems and never inflict them on other people. The CENTUARY type, persons who are easily influenced, are the special victims of the HEATHER folk, for the former have not the strength of will nor the wisdom to get up and walk away from them. The HEATHER type can completely deplete the MIMULUS people also, for the latter are too nervous and lacking in courage to make the break.

The description above is of the HEATHER type person. Yet, there are times when most of us suffer from the same state of mind, when we feel the need to talk about ourselves and our problems, even though we know that we may be boring our friendly listeners. This is because we ourselves are depleted, and our troubles become magnified and seem insurmountable. The HEATHER Remedy will soon restore our vitality, and we shall be our normal selves once again.

The positive qualities of HEATHER are found in the selfless, understanding individual who has suffered so greatly himself that he is very willing to listen to and help others. Such a person can put his own difficulties behind him and become absorbed in the problems of others. He is unsparing in his efforts to help them.

CASE HISTORIES

This is an excerpt from a letter of the friend of a patient: "She is staying with us at present. She appears terribly self-centered and selfish. She cannot get away from herself for long, and she talks all the time about her aches and pains. This morning she told me at length that she had written a letter the night before and it had tired her so much that she expected to have a headache all the day. The curtains were drawn in her room, and she had a shade over her eyes, but she had no headache!" When we saw that patient, she gave a long and detailed account of her symptoms both past and present. She said that she lived a very lonely life because few people came to see her, and when they did, they would never stay long enough to listen to all of her troubles, or give her the sympathy she needed. HEATHER the type Remedy was prescribed, and there was an immediate improvement during the first three weeks. She began gradually to take interest in things around her. She made friends with a very busy woman whom she helped with her children, the shopping and in her home. Her health had improved beyond measure, and after another month, she suffered from no further ailments.

Boy, age 17. He was about to take his examinations for the University. He was a bright student who enjoyed his studies and was also good at athletics. However, for the past year he had been continually worrying about himself. He worried about the examinations, his future, his health, until finally he all but exhausted his family with his problems. He began to have palpitations and insomnia and he had to tell everybody about his troubles. Consequently he began to lose friends. HEATHER the type Remedy was prescribed with good results. He became more carefree and joined in cycling excursions with his friends again; they enjoyed his company. In spite of these gains, he remained nervous about the forthcoming examinations. MIMULUS was added to the type Remedy to allay his anxiety. Within two weeks he reported that he felt much less nervous and was sleeping better. The palpitations had evidently disappeared, since he made no mention of them. He concluded by saying that he was sure he would be successful with his examinations, and indeed he was.

Woman, age 65. She was retired, and completely absorbed in her own troubles. She disliked being alone, and she was continually anticipating disaster. HEATHER was prescribed for her self-absorption; ASPEN for her fears of unknown origin. She took these Remedies for about six weeks. She then reported that she had lost not only her unfounded anxieties, but most of her imaginary ailments as well.

Man, age 57. The year before coming to us, he had a nervous breakdown, and in spite of various treatments, he had not recovered from it. He was prone to talk about his various symptoms and to give full details about his abnormal appetite, his constipation, his piles, and his mental and physica fatigue. HEATHER the type Remedy was prescribed for his self-concern; OLIVE for his fatigue and exhaustion. Although he felt better after the first month, he remained quite despairing about ever being cured; GORSE was added to the Remedies to correct this condition. The result was immediate; he felt much better and started to do some part-time work. The Remedies were repeated, but changed from time to time as his state of mind changed; HEATHER the type Remedy was always included. After six months he reported that he was completely cured, and that he was most grateful.

Man, age 60, a gardener. He was a great talker who would buttonhole his friends in the street and tell them all about himself, his ailments, and his past life *ad nauseam*. He sapped the energy of those whom he could persuade to listen to him. Though he lived alone, he much preferred to be with people all of the time. He suffered from varicose veins, frequent colds, constipation and a rash on his hands. HEATHER the type Remedy was prescribed for his self-concern. He took the Remedy over a long period of time. Eventually, he was greatly helped physically, but the change in his state of mind was notable. He became interested in the problems of others, and helped them in many ways. He was greatly liked in his village.

Woman, age 59, a housekeeper. She talked incessantly about one of the boarders in the house where she worked. Her attitude toward him amounted to an obsession, and she related how he interfered with her work, and even sought to destroy the pleasant relations she enjoyed with her employer. Each time that she came to see us, she gave an account in detail of every occurrence, repeating her stories time after time. Consumed with deep resentment, she blamed the boarder for the deterioration in her health. She had a painful and chronic ulcer on her left ankle which troubled her greatly and refused to heal. HEATHER the type Remedy was prescribed for her excessive self-preoccupation; WILLOW for her great resentment. She was instructed to take these orally, and an ointment for the ulcer was prepared as well. The treatment was continued for more than a year. At the end of that time, the ulcer had healed completely and it never recurred; but the greatest change took place within herself. She had become a most understanding person, sympathetic toward the point of view of others, and entirely free of any resentment.

Woman, age 48, married. She was a huge woman, greatly overweight at about 175 pounds. She never ceased talking about her physical complaints, which were many. Some of these were: pains around the eyes; pain over the forehead; cramps at night; frequent head colds; choking and vomiting; sores on her nose and lips; hot flushes, and many other ailments too numerous to mention. She owned a shop, and so had a ready-made audience in her customers. She feared loneliness and felt a constant need to be with other people. HEATHER was given for her compulsion to talk about herself; CRAB APPLE to cleanse her mind and body. After she had taken the Remedies for six months, she showed a remarkable improvement in her health. She had lost weight, and all of her miseries had vanished! Much to her surprise, she found that being without people around her did not make her feel lonesome. In fact she "got away from it all" by taking her dogs for long walks in the country.

CHAPTER 16

HOLLY

Keywords: Hatred; envy; jealousy; suspicion

HOLLY could well be the most important of all the Remedies, for it is the antidote for hatred! Hatred can be considered as the fundamental cause of every difficulty in life, because it is the antithesis of love, and love is the greatest force in the world, for God is love. Hatred lies behind all the negative aspects of the human character. It is impossible to be afraid, jealous, intolerant or depressed if one truly loves, and feels oneself loved, for "perfect love casts out all fear". Hatred is the absence of love, as darkness is the absence of light. It separates one from God and man. Hatred breeds insecurity, aggressiveness, jealousy, envy and suspicion; it produces feelings of misunderstanding, bad-temper and anger toward one's fellow man, because it is contrary to the Unity of Being. Dr. Bach said: "HOLLY protects us from everything that is not Universal Love." Dr. Bach also made an observation about the empirical use of HOLLY and WILD OAT when a case does not respond well to the Remedies prescribed: "If ever a case suggests that it needs many Remedies, or if ever a case does not respond to treatment, give either HOLLY or WILD OAT, and it will then be obvious which other Remedies may be required. In all cases where the patient is of the active, intense type, give HOLLY. In patients who are of the weak, despondent type, give WILD OAT."

The positive aspects of HOLLY are seen in those people who can give without wanting anything in return; in those who can be loving, tolerant and happy, although they may have lost everything; in those who can rejoice to see others take their rightful place. Such persons can bear the vexations of life with understanding and tolerance.

CASE HISTORIES

Child, age 3. He felt that his new little sister was receiving all of the attention, and that he had to play by himself. To attract attention, he began to pinch and push the baby and make her cry. When he was scolded, he would throw himself on the floor and kick and scream. HOLLY the type Remedy was prescribed for the child's jealousy. Within a few weeks there had been a definite change in his attitude and actions towards his little sister. He became so happy that his mother had to caution him against singing too loudly and waking the baby.

Man, age 65, widower, a retired army Colonel. Seven years before we saw him, he had a cancer of the throat which had been successfully operated on, and up to this time, had not recurred. The Colonel was very devoted to his only daughter. Although he liked her fiancé, whom she planned to marry soon, he dreaded the thought of her leaving home. He became ill. In order to play upon his daughter's sympathy, he would not eat, and he complained of his throat continually. He also developed a jealous and intense dislike for his daughter's fiancé. His attitude caused his daughter great distress; she was torn between her duty toward her father, and her love for her fiancé. Her father refused to see a doctor, because he feared that the cancer might have returned. He was referred to us for treatment. HOLLY was prescribed for his jealous attitude toward the young man; CHICORY for his possessive attitude towards his daughter. One month later, the fiancé wrote to us and said: "The

Colonel has made great strides in the right direction. He now joins us in discussions about the forthcoming wedding. He is much more like his old self. He is eating better, and altogether he has made a remarkable recovery." His daughter says that "it is simply amazing." The Remedies were continued for another month. The Colonel gave his daughter in marriage and wished the young couple great happiness. Since then he has been eating well, and has not complained about his throat.

Man, middle age. When he applied to us for treatment, he had a severe rash on his arms and hands. He was a hate-filled man of violent temper, and had become depressed and fatigued in his work which he thoroughly disliked. HOLLY was prescribed for his strong hatred; OLIVE for his fatigue and lack of interest; CRAB APPLE to cleanse him from the toxins of hatred which caused the rash. Within two months, he wrote to say: "I am so much better in every way; I sleep well and I have regained an interest in my work. I have become much more tolerant of my fellow workers. The rash has disappeared, although at times there is a little irritation." One month later, he wrote to say that the irritation had disappeared entirely, and that he felt normal and well.

The following extract is from a letter written to us by a wife, about her husband: "My husband has been a deep-sea diver for thirty years. He worked on unexploded bombs and shells in Plymouth Harbour during the war. He retired seven years ago. These deep-sea divers all become ill due to breathing compressed air whilst they are working in the dark on the sea-bed. It makes them hard and cruel, as it did my husband, who is by nature a kind and generous man. Now, he is silent, and tormented by hatred. He has no feelings of compassion for anyone who is in trouble or who is ill. He is of course a very brave man, but he is filled with self-pity and speaks of himself as 'poor me' quite frequently. He suffers from claustrophobia, and he keeps all of the doors and windows in the house open, even in winter. He is always restless, and cannot stop moving about, and he is very unsociable." HOLLY was prescribed for the hatred and hardness which was against his nature; CHICORY for his self-pity; MIMULUS for his fear of closed places. Within six months, he responded excellently. First he overcame the claustrophobia, and he could remain in the house with the doors and the windows closed. He became much calmer and happier and so pleasant that finally his family wrote to say: "He has changed so very much that we all love him, and like to be with him."

Woman, age 73, a widow. She wrote to us saying: "I get suddenly exhausted as if I had nothing at all inside me. I think that it is due to my nasty thoughts. I am discontented and not counting my blessings. I really hate my neighbor who has such a happy life." HOLLY was given to overcome her jealousy; OLIVE for the fatigue. Two months later she was a different woman. The fatigue had left, and she wrote to say: "I am making a friend of my neighbor. I have found out that she is such a nice woman, and so understanding."

CHAPTER 17

HONEYSUCKLE

Keywords: Dwelling upon thoughts of the past; nostalgia; homesickness

DR. BACH wrote of HONEYSUCKLE: "This is the Remedy to remove from the mind the regrets and sorrows of the past, to counteract all influences, all wishes and desires of the past and to bring us back into the present. Living in the past, as a state of mind, does not occur only in the aged, though it is but natural that their thoughts should return to pleasant memories of years gone by and the friends and experiences of their youth." It also can be seen in the homesick youngster during his first days at school or away from home, for he too dwells in the past, though the past is not far removed in time. During any period of unhappiness, boredom or sorrow, the mind may revert to the memory of a lost friend, or to ambitions which were never fulfilled. Under those conditions an individual may lose interest in the present, and he may make no effort to confront existing difficulties; the body is left to struggle on in the present moment, while the mind relives the past and does not contribute to the well-being of the body. This causes an inharmonious state of near-stagnation, a definite slowing down of the vital life forces. It has well been called the "state of Lot's wife", for while the mind is looking backward with fear, longing, or sadness, the body is being consumed by the fire of the present, and remains petrified in regard to the life which lies ahead.

A typical example is that of a soldier who, after the war suffered from nervousness, depression and panic because he could not forget his experiences in the Battle of Crete. Another example is the patient who said: "When my husband died, half of me died too." The Remedy HONEYSUCKLE also is prescribed for nostalgia: a patient wrote: "We have moved into another district. How I wish that we had never moved! I have found out that I was happy where I was." There is a resemblance between HONEYSUCKLE and CLEMATIS types, for neither is fully alive in the present moment; the CLEMATIS state of mind is a dreamy one with the hope of a better future, while that of HONEYSUCKLE lives in the past and holds a pessimistic outlook both for the present and the future.

The positive aspect of HONEYSUCKLE is clearly seen in those persons who retain the lesson taught by past experiences, while allowing the experience itself to pass out of their mind.

CASE HISTORIES

Woman, age 50. When she was a small child, her drunken father had threatened to choke her, and ever since she had suffered from the fear of choking and suffocation. The onset of the climacteric had increased these fears, and she began to feel that her throat was closing up. An X-ray examination showed no physical cause for the sensation. Although she was cheerful and kind by nature, she nevertheless felt a deep resentment toward her father. HONEYSUCKLE was prescribed as the type Remedy, to counteract the childhood memories; HOLLY for the resentment she felt towards her father; ROCK ROSE for her great fear of suffocation. Within three weeks she was able to report that she could swallow normally and that she had lost the sensation of having a tight band around her throat. Two months later she wrote to say that she neither resented her father, nor did she dwell upon the unpleasant memories of her childhood any more; she did say however that her throat never bothered her unless she was overtired.* One month later, all symptoms had disappeared, and a friend of hers wrote to say: "I have never seen such a change in anyone in such a short time."

Woman, middle age, a widow. Her husband had died three years before she applied to us for treatment. After his death, she began to suffer from periodic and severe attacks of colitis. She wrote: "I am so depressed, and I miss my husband so much. I feel that there is no more interest left in life." HONEYSUCKLE was prescribed for her thoughts of the past, and loss of interest in the present; STAR OF BETHLEHEM to counteract the shock of her husband's death, even though his illness had been one of long duration. Her first report indicated that she was less depressed and that the colitis had ceased to trouble her; she seemed to have gained more interest in life, and more vitality. She continued to take the Remedies for another three months, when she wrote again to say that she was cheerful, and that she was working; her stomach trouble had not returned.

Woman, middle age, a nurse by profession. When she applied to us for treatment, she was very tired, and felt depressed. She liked her work at a County Hospital, but for some years she suffered from catarrh. During her conversation with us, it was discovered that while she was a probationer at the same hospital, she would become very nervous when the doctors made their rounds. She remembered that she always had to blow her nose, and to clear her throat. HONEYSUCKLE was prescribed, because we felt that the memory of those days still persisted in spite of the fact that she was now an experienced and efficient nurse; CRAB APPLE was added as a cleanser of the mind and body. Much to her surprise, the catarrh which had been termed chronic, cleared up within three weeks, and never returned to trouble her again!

---

* Dr. Bach always said: "Never get overtired, never get cold, and never go hungry." These are conditions which affect the psychic system; especially in a patient under treatment.

Woman, age 40, a widow. Three years before she came to us for treatment, her husband had been hit by a truck, and was fatally injured. She nursed him until his death. Shortly after that, she herself suffered a fall, and although there were no broken bones, one of her legs continued to ache. The pain seemed to be most severe whenever her thoughts turned back to her husband's illness and death. She told us that she was lonely and that she missed him greatly, and thoughts of their happy years together would often enter her mind. She was depressed, she suffered from continual headaches, and she was sleeping badly. HONEYSUCKLE was the Remedy indicated for the thoughts of the past; STAR OF BETHLEHEM for the long lasting shock of her husband's death; CHICORY for the effects of self-pity. The next month she reported that she felt much better and that she was brighter in spirit; she had much less pain in her leg. She continued the Remedies for another two months, when she wrote to say that she was now fine; she was sleeping well again, she had no headaches, and all of the pain had left her leg. The following year she wrote to say that there had been no relapse, and that she was happily re-married.

Man, age 46. His job called for long hours of tedious but light work. The year before, he had a failure in business, and as he said: "The memory of that keeps returning very often." He was tired and depressed, and he suffered from indigestion. HONEYSUCKLE was prescribed for the memories of the past; GENTIAN for the depression. Emotionally, he responded well to the Remedies, but he complained that they gave him a rash on his chest. It was evident that the Remedies were giving his system a thorough cleansing! CRAB APPLE was added, and the rash quickly disappeared. After a long period of time, he wrote to say that none of the symptoms had returned.

Man, middle age, a placid person by nature. He told us that he had lost his temper only once during fifteen years of married life! He complained that he tossed about in his sleep, and that he had troublesome dreams which he could not recall. What he could remember concerned being confined in a small space, and trying to fight his way out; this was an actual experience from his childhood. His situation was aggravated by the fact that the ship in which he had been serving in the Korean war was hit by a bomb; he had been blown to the deck below, and badly injured. HONEYSUCKLE was prescribed to help him forget the events of the past; AGRIMONY was his type Remedy, and that was added also. The next month he wrote to say that he had been sleeping better, and had only three disturbed nights since he started the treatment. After another two months, he could write that he felt fine; that he was again sleeping deeply and peacefully, and that he was perfectly happy.

Woman, age 60. She was referred to us by a physician. She lived completely in the past, and wept and fretted about her relatives who had died. She talked incessantly about them, and of the happy times they had spent together. HONEYSUCKLE the type Remedy was prescribed. The effect was immediate, and remarkable. She recovered completely within one week.

Woman, age 40. During the past years when she had been visiting with relatives, twice she had been called to help a sudden illness in the night. Now she found that whenever she was in a strange house she would awaken in fear, and it took her some time before she could go back to sleep again. HONEYSUCKLE was prescribed, because it was believed that the fear was what might be called "a memory fear"; MIMULUS was added to allay any actual fear that might come upon her. Within two months she wrote to say: "The Remedies have been most successful. I spent Christmas with relatives, and I have been away on visits quite a number of times since then, and I have slept well every night."

CHAPTER 18

HORNBEAM

Keywords: Tiredness; weariness; mental and physical exhaustion

THE weariness for which we prescribe HORNBEAM is, properly speaking, a fatigue that asserts itself more in the mind than in the body. There are times when a person is assailed by the doubt that he has sufficient strength or ability to face either life or his work; yet in spite of that, he usually accomplished the task without difficulty. At these times, HORNBEAM will fortify him mentally and physically. In convalescence it helps those patients who question whether they have the physical strength to use their limbs, or to walk; it also helps those who feel that they do not have sufficient mental energy to return to work. In health, this Remedy gives "backbone" to those who feel weary in mind and body. There are those who say: "I feel more tired getting up in the morning than when I go to bed", or "I often feel that I cannot cope with the things and ideas that I have to deal with at the moment." HORN-BEAM is the Remedy for such people. Somebody described HORNBEAM most aptly as "The Monday morning Remedy"; indeed it is the Remedy for the "morning after" feeling! HORNBEAM differs from the weakness of the OLIVE state of mind in that the latter is the result of great mental and physical suffering or the debility brought about by long illness. The HORNBEAM tiredness on the other hand is a fatigue which often

116

passes away when the individual becomes interested in his normal activities, and takes his mind off himself.

The positive aspect of HORNBEAM is reflected in those who are certain of their own ability and strength, even though their work might appear to be beyond their capacities to achieve.

CASE HISTORIES

Woman, age 53, unmarried. She was the Headmistress of a girls' school, and was working under a great strain. Every morning she would wake up feeling so tired that she felt she would not be able to get through the day's work. So intense was this feeling that she was considering resigning her position. Her eyes were giving her much trouble as well. HORNBEAM was prescribed for the general feeling of tiredness; SCLERANTHUS to help her come to a definite decision, for the indecision was contributing to her emotional distress. Improvement was rapid and definite. She reported that she felt less fatigued, and that the eyestrain had decreased. She continued the treatment for three months. At the end of that time she wrote to say: "I am feeling very well again, and my eyes trouble me only occasionally. Once again I have the energy and the ability to carry out my work, and I do not procrastinate as I used to do."

Woman, age 50, married. She had become very irritable and snappish, and she wondered whether she had the strength to continue to look after her married daughter who was expecting a baby in two weeks time. She did not feel that she could face the extra work her daughter's presence demanded. Normally she was active and energetic, but now although she still managed to do her housework, the very thought of it tired her. She had developed sores between her toes, open cracks which distressed her greatly. HORNBEAM was prescribed for the fatigue of mind and body; IMPATIENS for her irritability. Within three weeks she wrote to say: "The medicine has acted like a miracle. I have become a different creature within a few days! The baby has arrived and all went happily and merrily! The toes are healing nicely." She wrote again in another month and said that she was really well again, and that the condition of her toes had cleared up completely.

Man, middle age, an Air Chief Marshal in the R.A.F. He had been overworking, driving himself too hard for several years. He now awoke in the mornings and felt that he would never be able to face his day's work, although somehow he always was able to do it. He was suffering from varicose veins, and that made standing difficult for him; an operation was urged, but he wanted to try the Bach Remedies first. HORNBEAM was prescribed to give him strength and vitality for his work; it was also given to him as a lotion with which to bathe his legs. He followed the treatment for some weeks with good results. Now when he awakened in the morning, he once again looked forward to the work of the day. After three months more of the treatment, he found that he could stand for long periods of time without discomfort, and the swelling of the veins had subsided almost entirely, much to the surprise of the surgeon! He was completely cured and no operation was necessary. The condition did not return.

Woman, middle age, single. She stated that she was always very tired. When she awoke in the morning, she felt as if she could not get out of bed, and that she would never be able to get her housework done. Her sleep was disturbed by night-mares. The year before, she had been in a major train acci-dent, and while she had not been injured, she suffered greatly from shock and was now frightened of trains. Al-though she had started to feel tired before the accident, she believed that if she could overcome the fatigue, all of her other fears would disappear. HORNBEAM was prescribed for the fatigue; STAR OF BETHLEHEM for the shock of the train accident; HONEYSUCKLE to counteract the memory of the wreck. The Remedies were also made up as a lotion which she applied to her left hand which was painful and swollen from a domestic accident. Within a month she reported to us that she had taken a train to Edinburgh, and that much to her surprise, she had not been as nervous as she expected to be. She added that she felt better and more rested. The Remedies were repeated, with the addition of CRAB APPLE because she had a discharge from her right eye; an eye specialist had told her that nothing but an operation could cure the condition. Her next report was very good; her eye was well, and the specialist now declared that an operation was not needed. The pain in her hand had at first increased, but now had vanished altogether. She was cured, and she had no recurrence.

Man, age 62. He had lost his right arm as the result of an accident while at work. Recently he had been sleeping badly; he felt very weak, and doubted whether he could continue to work. He was also suffering from indigestion and from a depression which at times reached the point of utter hopelessness. HORNBEAM was prescribed to strengthen his mind and body; GORSE for the feeling of hopelessness. The response was rapid and notable. Within the first month he wrote: "I feel my old self again. My appetite is good, and I am eating well and am suffering no ill effects. I sleep well and restfully all night through."

Woman, age 29, married. She was a professional ballet dancer. At the time she applied to us, she awakened each morning tired mentally and physically, and wondered whether she would be able to do her strenuous day's work; she was beginning to think that it was beyond her ability. She suffered from constipation and visceroptosis which caused intense pain after each meal. In consequence, she went without food as often as she could, and this contributed toward her tiredness and weakness. She had an abnormal fear of becoming ill, because as a child her mother had always become very angry when she was sick. HORNBEAM was prescribed for her tired mind and body; MIMULUS for her fear of illness; GENTIAN for her depression and despair. Within the first ten days of the treatment, she began to feel better. She did not have the pain after eating as regularly as before, but she still had to force herself to face the day. The Remedies were repeated, and she continued to take them for another three months. Her condition improved gradually. The constipation disappeared, and she had regular movements each day. She was completely free of pain after eating. She continued to take the Remedies, and some months thereafter she wrote: "I feel wonderfully well! I have no bad news to report! I am so much stronger, and I am filled with vitality."

Woman, age 40, a widow. She had lost her husband some three and a half years before coming to us. Since his death, she said that she felt fatigued in mind and body; that she could hardly face each day as it arrived. One year previously, she had experienced violent pains in the abdomen; these would come and go; sometimes they lasted as long as six weeks at a time. Recently, they had begun to recur with increasing frequency, until finally, when she came to us, she had developed a severe colitis with diarrhea. She said that the pain started before she got up in the morning, and that pre-scribed diets made no difference; she took liquids only, and had lost much weight because of the continuous diarrhea. HORNBEAM was prescribed to give her strength; MIMULUS because of fear of the violent pains and the frequent bowel actions; SCLERANTHUS because she said that she was unable to make up her mind about anything. After one month, she said: "I feel brighter and stronger, but the diarrhea and the pains are still there." Two months later she wrote again to say: "I am feeling ever so much better. I am not nearly so distressed, and I am much more ready to get up in the morn-ings and get on with my work. The pains and the diarrhea have not occurred for the past month." She continued the Remedies for another month, but neither the pains nor the diarrhea returned.

CHAPTER 19

IMPATIENS

Keywords: Impatience; irritability; extreme mental tension

THIS is the Remedy for those people who are quick in mind and action. It is for those who make instant decisions and like to work alone because the slowness of others might hinder them. They grasp any new idea or subject quickly, and they may sometimes finish a sentence if the speaker is slow; at times they might even snatch things out of another person's hands if he is not quick enough to suit them. They are active people and nervous; they move, eat and speak quickly. They are intelligent and intuitive, good and efficient in whatever they undertake. They tend to become impatient and sometimes irritable with those who are not as quick as they are, but their anger which flares up quickly, just as quickly subsides. When these people are ill, they never feel that they are recovering fast enough, and they become irritated and impatient with both the situation and those around them. The extreme mental tension often manifests itself as muscular tension and pain. The IMPATIENS type is accident prone; they may well cross the street without a look at the approaching traffic and get stuck by an automobile, or they may run blindly ahead, not seeing obstacles in their path. Thus they get injured through their own impetuousness. When they are in a bad temper, they are also prone to do things brusquely, such as slamming a door on their fingers, or jerking a boiling kettle from the stove and burning themselves. IMPATIENS is an effective Remedy for all manifestations of pain caused by tension such as a sudden cramp, an agonizing pain, or other spastic condition. The IMPATIENS type may also suffer from indigestion and allied complaints brought about by their irritable nature, for it is a fact that eating when one is emotionally or nervously upset affects the digestion directly. The IMPATIENS type differs from the VERVAIN type in that the latter person exhausts his vitality through over-use of effort and strong will and the IMPATIENS person becomes exhausted through frustration and nervous effort when things do not move fast enough. The IMPATIENS type prefers to work alone and unhindered, and when he is allowed to do so, he never tries to influence others as the VERVAIN type sometimes does.

The positive qualities of the IMPATIENS type are their great gentleness and sympathy towards others. They are capable, decisive, intuitive and clever, with abilities far above the average. At the same time they are understanding and tolerant with those who are slower than themselves.

CASE HISTORIES

Dr. Bach himself had found that this Remedy had a very quick acting effect. He had, of course, an intimate knowledge and an understanding of the Remedies and their possibilities. There were times when he was inclined to become impatient, when others were not as quick as he was, and were slow to follow his line of thought. When this occurred, he had an immediate physical reaction, and a red and very irritating rash would suddenly appear. He would say: "You see, my being irritable with you hurts me more than it hurts you!" A dose of IMPATIENS would restore his good humor, and within a short time the rash would disappear.

From the case records of F. J. Wheeler, M.B.: "Woman, age

60. She was always inclined to be in a hurry. She fell down some steps and sprained one ankle badly and the other slightly. The badly sprained ankle was bruised, stiff and swollen. IMPATIENS the type Remedy was prescribed both to be taken internally, and applied as a lotion. The patient had a good night, without discomfort, and the next day the ankle was much better. Treatment was continued until the ankle showed no sign of the accident."

Woman, age 24, married and a mother. She suffered intense pain each month during the menstrual period. A pelvic examination revealed that she had an ulcer. An operation was advised, and she was told to return in one month for another examination. The woman was terrified of the operation, and during the attacks of pain, she became hysterical at the thought of it. By nature she was capable, quick and efficient, but resentful of interference or advice. IMPATIENS the type Remedy was prescribed for her quick and impatient nature; ROCK ROSE for the terror and panic; STAR OF BETHLEHEM for the shock that the prospect of an operation had caused. She took the medicine regularly for one month. Her next period was a mild one, with very little pain. When she returned to the hospital for the second examination, the surgeon was surprised to find no trace of the ulcer whatsoever; only a scar remained to show that there had been one. No operation was necessary.

Woman, age 40, married. She was a writer and had three children. By nature she was quick and impatient, and rather slapdash in her ways. She hated to waste energy or money, and she was begrudging of the time spent on her housework and away from her writing. When she came to us for treatment, she was suffering from an irritating rash on the fingers and palms of her hands. The rash appeared each spring, and this time it broke out with running ulcers on the palms. She felt unclean and was impatient about her cure. The children had been very trying to her during the winter, and this increased her tension to the point of insomnia. IMPATIENS the type Remedy was prescribed for her irritability and nervous tension; CRAB APPLE as a cleansing Remedy for mind and body. The Remedies were also made up as an ointment to be applied to her hands before bandaging them. The effects were remarkable, and fast. Within the first month, she wrote that her hands had healed with the exception of one finger, and that she was sleeping much better and could do her work once again. After another month, she was able to report that she was completely cured of the rash; she felt much better and she was not as irritable or cross with the children. Now, she said, they were a happy family group.

Woman, age 69. She was impatient and active by nature. When she applied to us for treatment, she was waiting her turn to go to a hospital for an operation. Though she had been under strain, and was tired, she said that she did not fear the operation. IMPATIENS was prescribed as the type Remedy; HORNBEAM to give her strength; MIMULUS because we felt that in spite of her statement to the contrary, she did have some fear of the operation. Her first report was that she felt amazingly well, and that she was much more hopeful about the future. She continued to take the Remedies until she went into the hospital. The operation was a success and she required a minimum of sedation. She was able to sleep every night without pills, and although she anticipated pain with the first bowel movement, the action was easy and comfortable. Her final letter to us said: "All is very well with me."

Woman, age 29, unmarried. She was a secretary and had been in the employ of the same firm for nine years. She was normally happy and full of life, quick, brilliant, but with a tendency to be impatient with others. She liked her work, but recently she stated that her employer had begun to nag her. He was always asking whether she was keeping things organized? Were the other girls doing their share of work? Couldn't she do more work? etc. The criticism was unjust and unnecessary and she became irritated and impatient because of it. She was fatigued and could not concentrate on her work. Her job was important to her, because she supported herself. IMPATIENS the type Remedy was prescribed for her quick and impatient nature; HORNBEAM to give her physical strength to overcome her difficulties. Within the first two weeks, she was able to say: "I feel soothed, and I am so happy, because I was really very upset." She continued to take the medicine for another month. At that time she said that she was her old self once more, and that she could listen to her employer's complaints without snapping back or even becoming irritated.

Extract from a letter received from a patient for whom we prescribed IMPATIENS. "Having taken the Remedy IMPATIENS for irritability for over a week, I am pleased to say that I am not so irritable as I was before I started, in spite of the fact that the cause of the irritation is exactly the same; some family trouble."

CHAPTER 20

LARCH

Keywords: Lack of confidence; anticipation of failure; despondency

LARCH is the Remedy for those people who have no confidence in themselves or in their abilities. They seldom attempt to do anything because they are sure they will fail. The LARCH type is not frightened as the MIMULUS people are; it is just that they are convinced they cannot do as well as others. This is unfortunate, because the LARCH type is as capable and as good as anyone else, and often superior. Here is an excerpt from a letter of a typical LARCH person. "Do you remember suggesting LARCH for my lack of self-confidence in the Dramatic Society? It helped me greatly, not only in that case but in many others! I find myself with much more determination, and I am now convinced that I shall do what I set out to do. My attitude towards my writing has undergone a great change. I never felt so determined before." Failure to even make the try leaves the LARCH type very despondent; one wrote: "I know that I shall never be a success, so I don't try. I feel inferior to other people, and that makes me despair." There is a certain false modesty in the admiration that the LARCH person shows for the success of others; they praise them and admire them without envy or jealousy. As a LARCH type wrote: "I often think why couldn't I have been like that or done things like he did? It is not envy on my part, just sort of wistfulness." Here is where they differ so greatly from the HOLLY state of mind which is based on jealousy and envy at another's success, and from the WILLOW outlook which is embittered and resentful at any failure. Shakespeare described the LARCH type perfectly when he wrote: "Our doubts are traitors and make us lose the good we oft might win by fearing to attempt."

The positive aspects of the LARCH character is reflected by the person who is willing to plunge into life; to take risks and never be discouraged by the results. Such a person knows that if he failed, it was not because he did not try his best. Such a one does not know the meaning of the word "can't".

CASE HISTORIES

Man, age 50. Since childhood he had always been self-conscious. He liked to be alone because he felt that he could not do as well as the other boys his age. Five years before he wrote us, he suffered a nervous breakdown. Now, in middle age, he felt that he was a failure. LARCH the type Remedy was prescribed for his lack of self-confidence; MIMULUS because of his fear of failure. After two months he wrote: "I can honestly say that I feel a great deal better than when I first wrote to you. I have a zest for life now, something that I never had before, and I am attempting to do many things that I have always wanted to do."

Boy, age 9. He was very unhappy at his school. He lacked confidence in everything he attempted, and worried himself into a state of nervous tension over the simple things that he thought he could not do. He feared swimming lessons, because he felt he was not as good at it as his companions were. For that reason he wanted to stay home every Tuesday, the day the swimming lessons were given. When his grandfather died, he became very upset emotionally, because he felt that he had lost understanding and support. LARCH the type

Remedy was prescribed for his lack of confidence; MIMULUS for his fear and nervousness; STAR OF BETHLEHEM for the shock of his grandfather's death. Within a month, his mother wrote to say: "You have no idea how much he has changed. He now loves swimming, and can hardly wait until Tuesday comes for his lesson. He is happy in his school now."

Children, it should be noted, respond very rapidly to the Remedies, and usually with excellent results. They do not resist the help the Remedies can give them, nor do they reason about them. Children simply want to get well and to be happy. Is there not an object lesson in this attitude?

Woman, middle age. She had never achieved the full success she was capable of, because since childhood she had lacked confidence in herself. She had always remained in a subordinate position because she was unable to take either initiative or responsibility. When she came to us, she suffered from a stiffness in her back, and became easily tired. The condition was chronic, and the treatment lasted over a long period of time, but finally her ailments were completely cured. The Remedies prescribed over this period were as follows: LARCH first, for some months until her confidence became such that she was able to break away from her subordinate position. She found a new position which required both initiative and enterprise, and demanded that she make her own decisions. OLIVE was then given, because at the start of her new work she became exhausted; WHITE CHESTNUT was added because she worried about her work. Progress continued to be slow but sure. She finally was able to report that she was well again, and that she had gained the respect and admiration of her associates.

Man, age 35. For the past eight years, he had been trying to pass his final examinations in medicine. He had taken the examinations three or four times a year, and he had always failed. He said: "I know that it is sheer examination nerves. I know my subject well." The last time that he went to London to take the examination, he was given LARCH for lack of confidence in himself; MIMULUS for his fear of failure. He

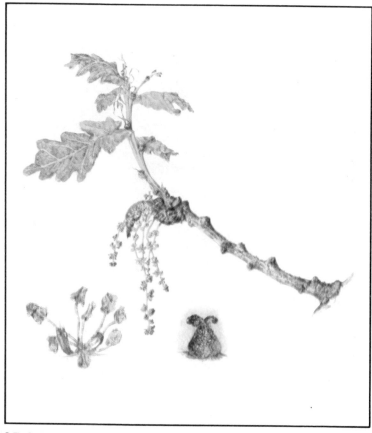

Oak—Quercus robur

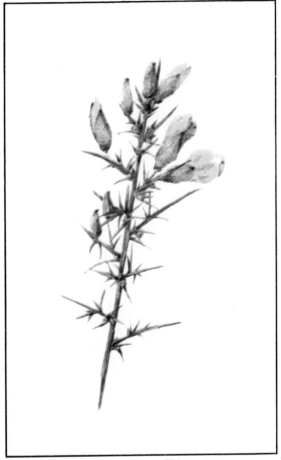

Gorse—Ulex europaeus

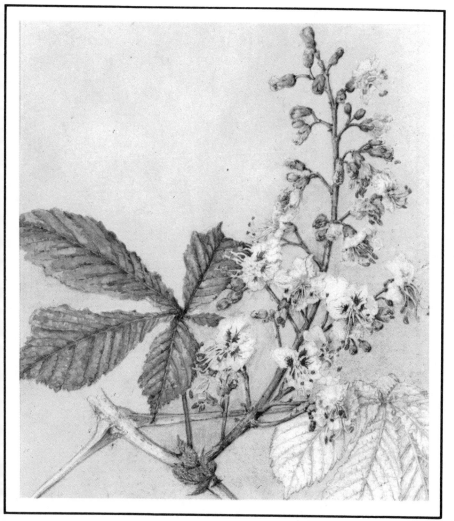

White Chestnut—Aesculus hippocastanum

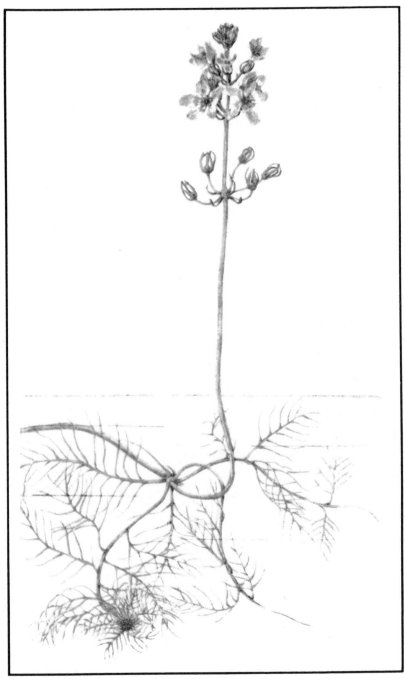

Water Violet—Hottonia palustris

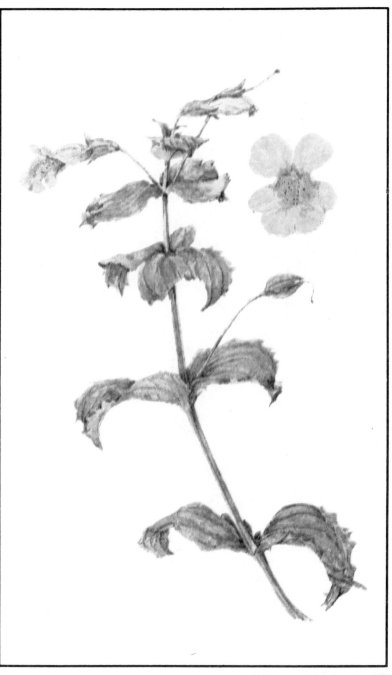

Mimulus—Mimulus *guttatus*

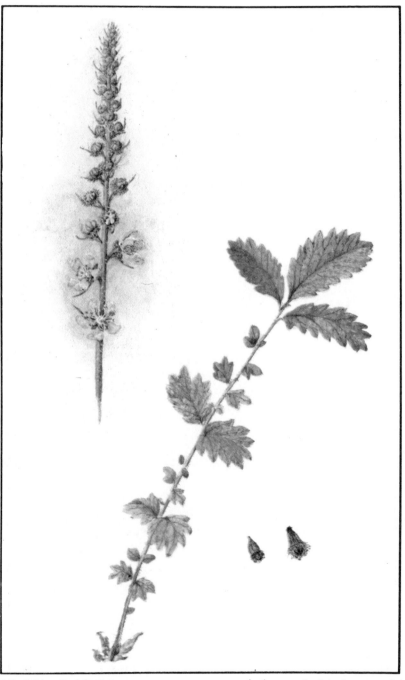

Agrimony—*Agrimonia eupatoria*

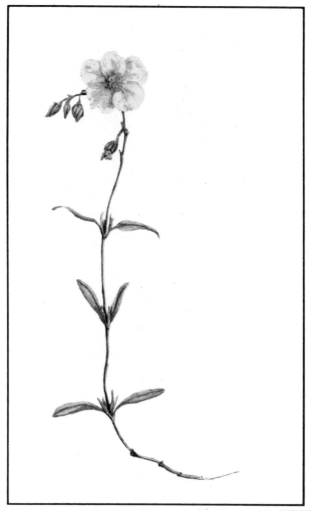

Rock Rose—Helianthemum nummularium

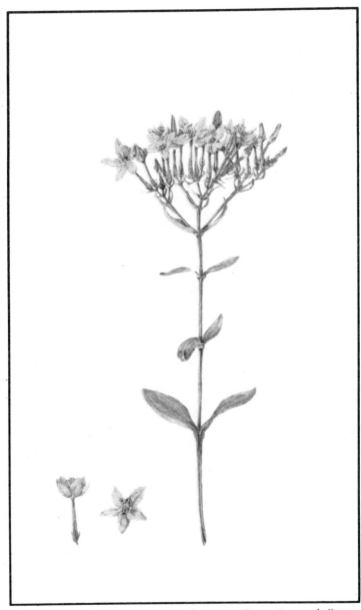

Centaury—Centaurium umbellatum

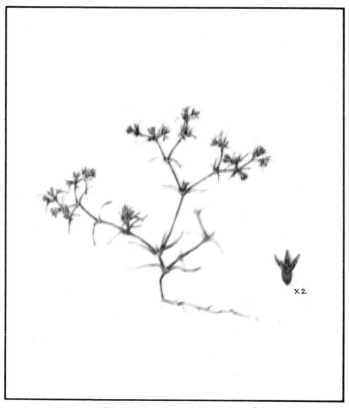

×2

Scleranthus—*Scleranthus annuus*

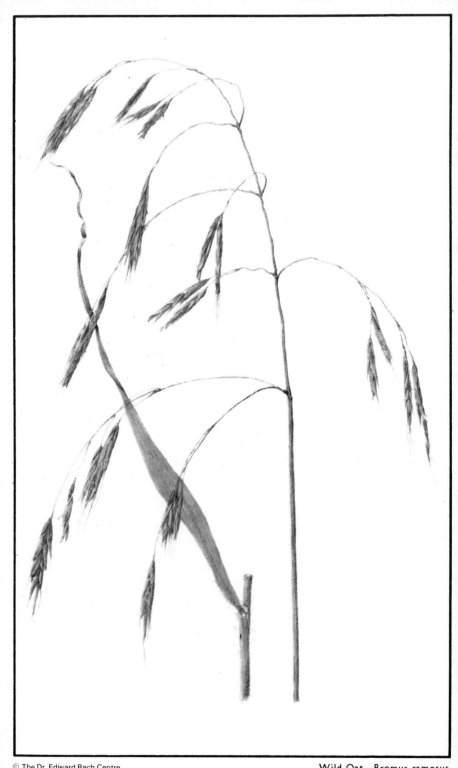

Wild Oat—Bromus ramosus

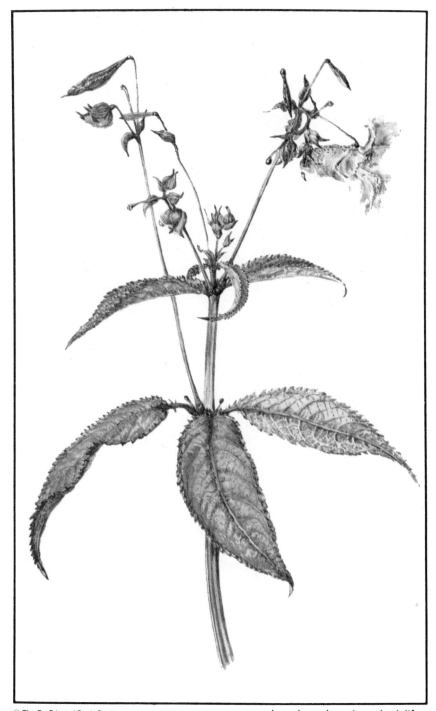

Impatiens—Impatiens glandulifera

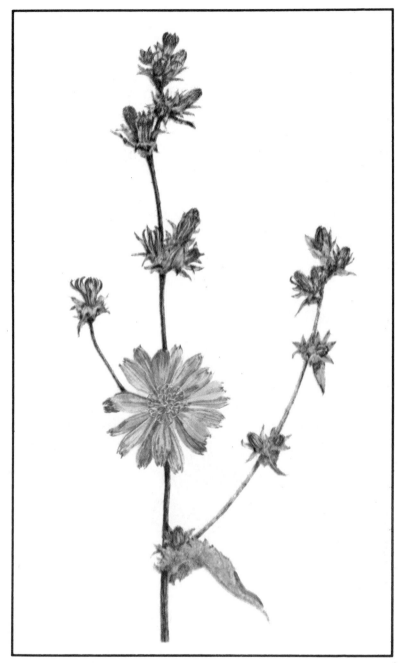

Chicory—Cichorium intybus

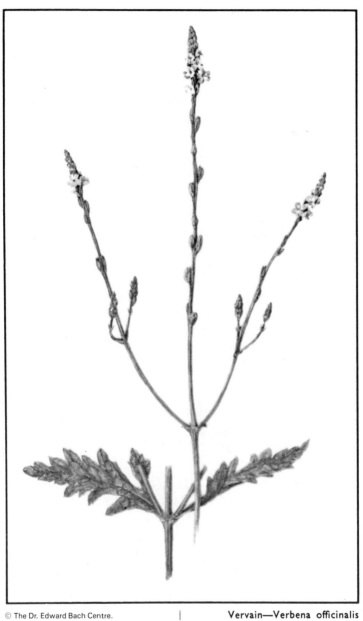

Vervain—Verbena officinalis

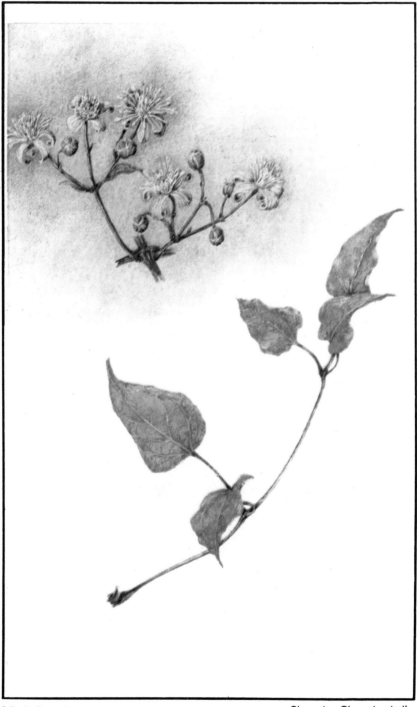

Clematis—Clematis vitalba

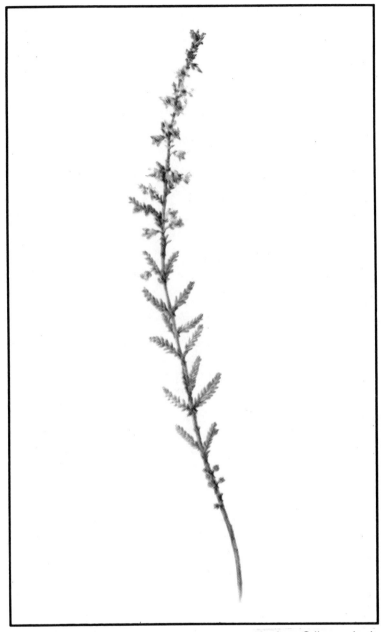

Heather—Calluna vulgaris

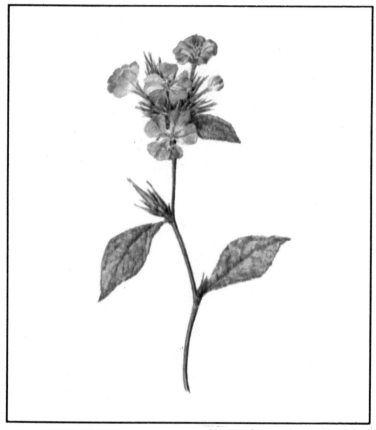

Cerato—Ceratostigma willmottiana

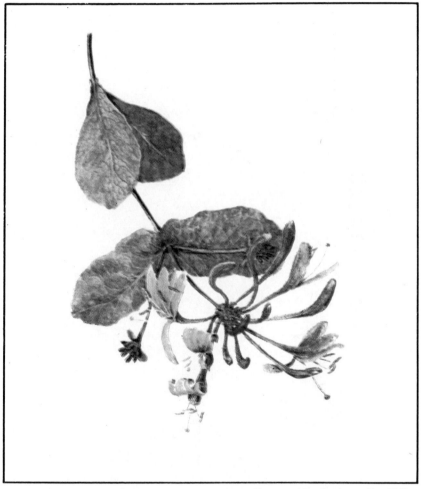

Honeysuckle—Lonicera Caprifolium

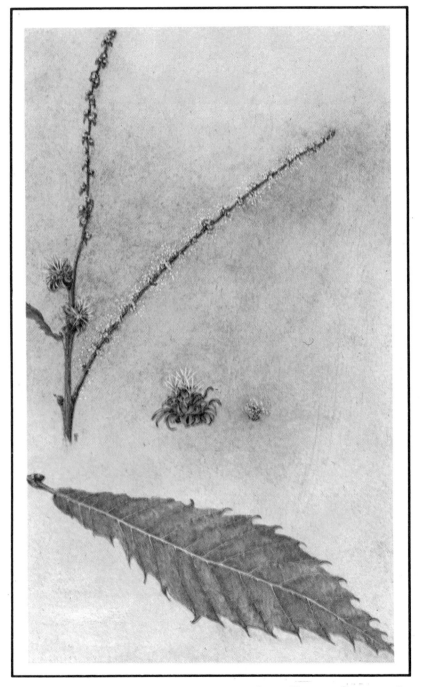

Sweet Chestnut—Castanea sativa

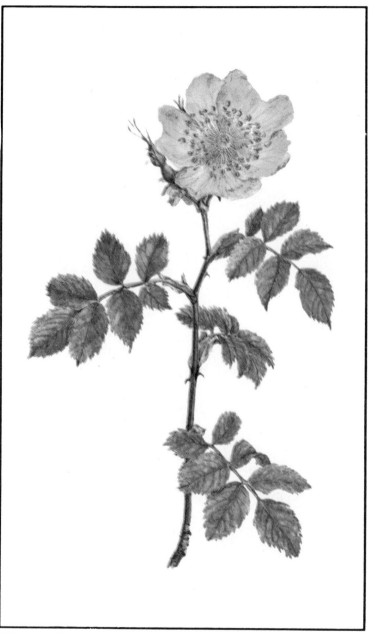

Wild Rose—Rosa canina

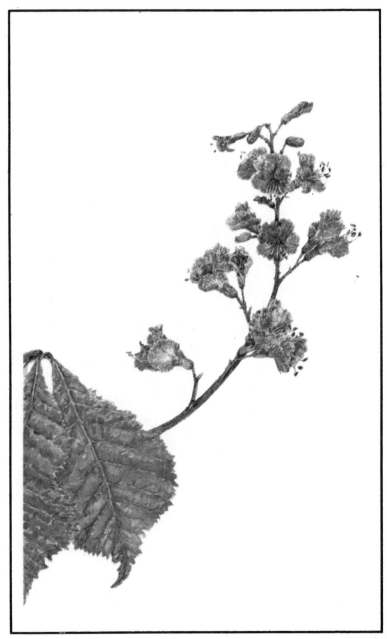

Red Chestnut—Aesculus carnea

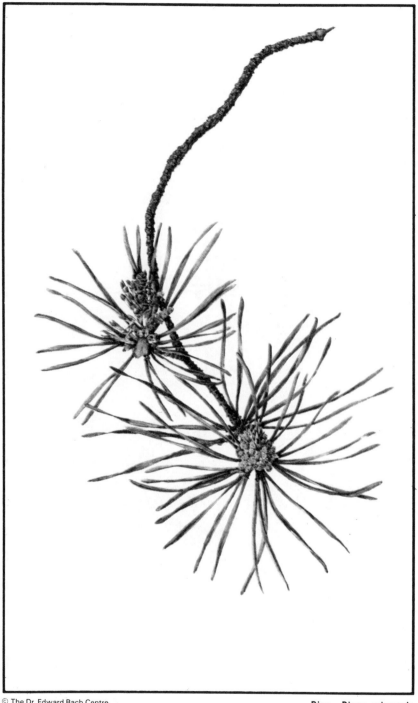

Pine—Pinus sylvestris

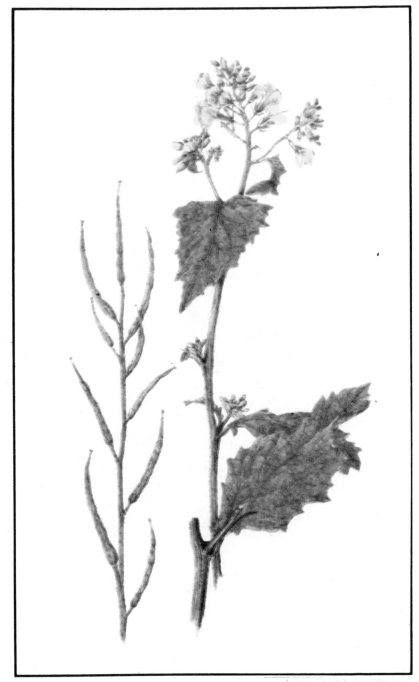

Mustard—Sinapis arvensis

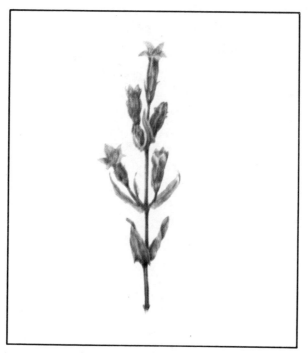

Gentian—*Gentiana amarella*

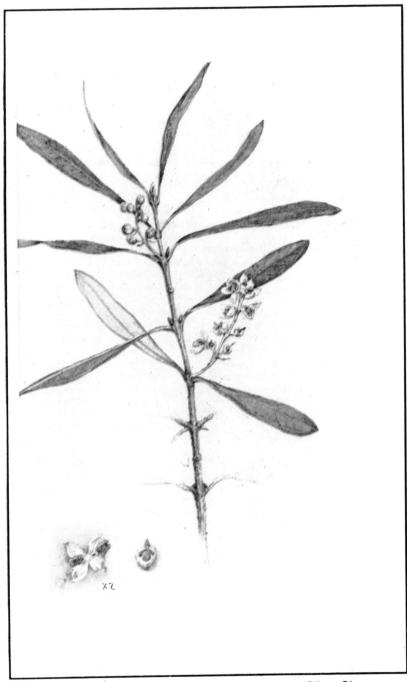

X2

Olive—Olea europaea

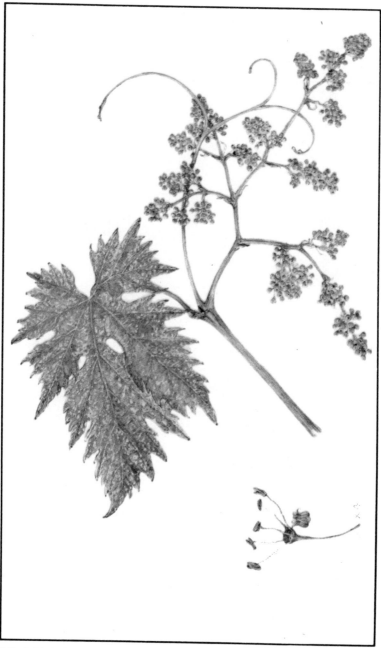

Vine—Vitis vinifera

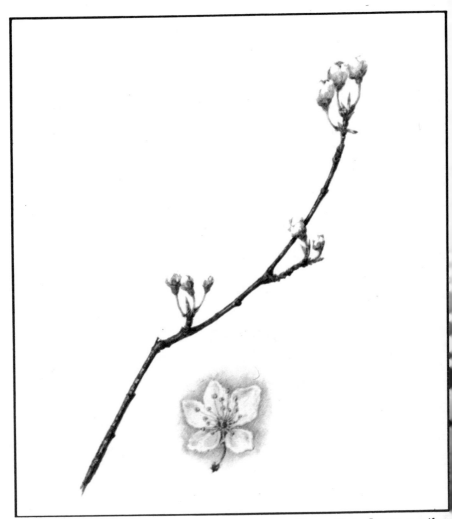

Cherry Plum—Prunus cerasifera

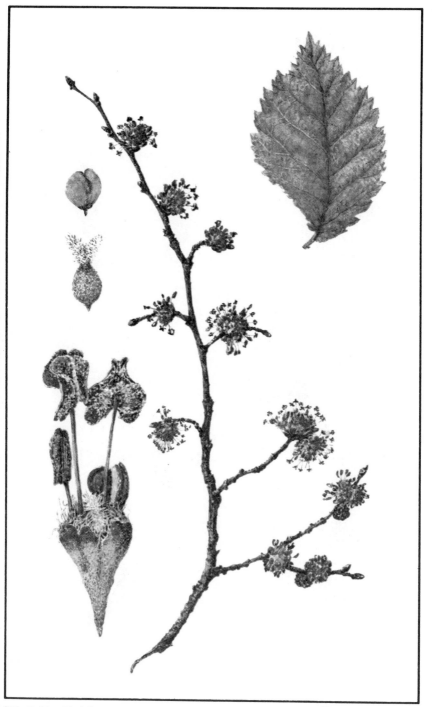

Elm—Ulmus procera

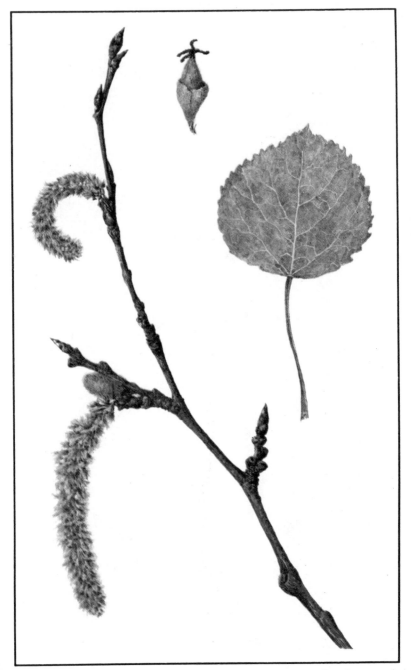

Aspen—Populus tremula

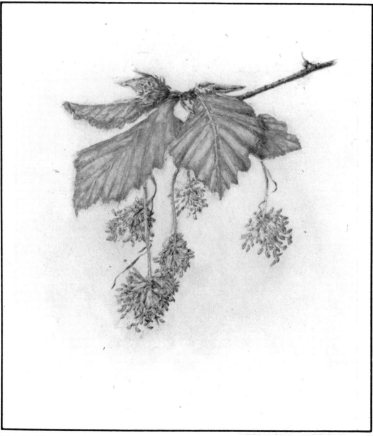

Beech—*Fagus sylvatica*

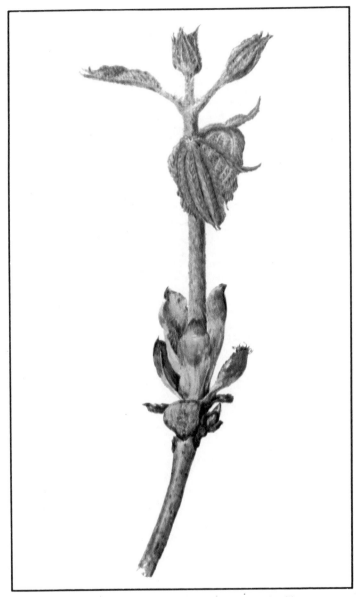

Chestnut Bud—Aesculus hippocastanum

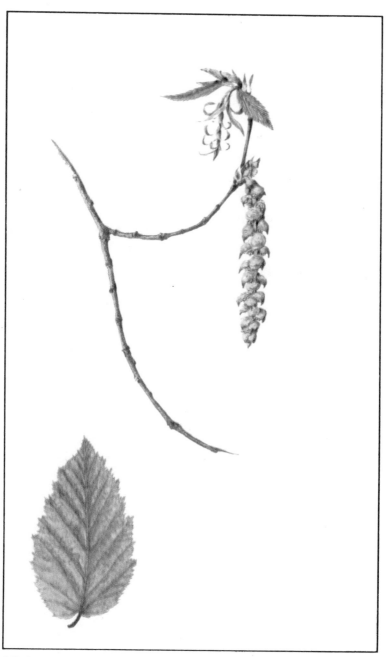

Hornbeam—Carpinus betulus

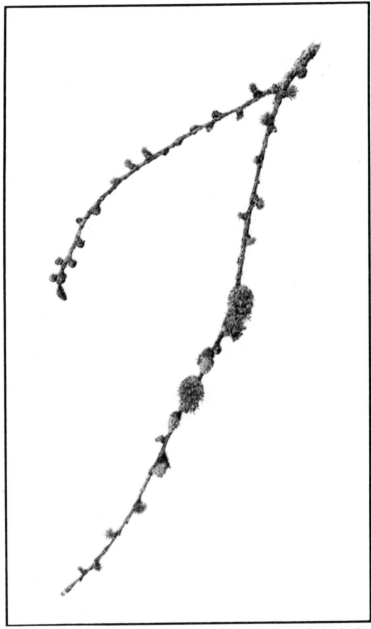

Larch—Larix decidua

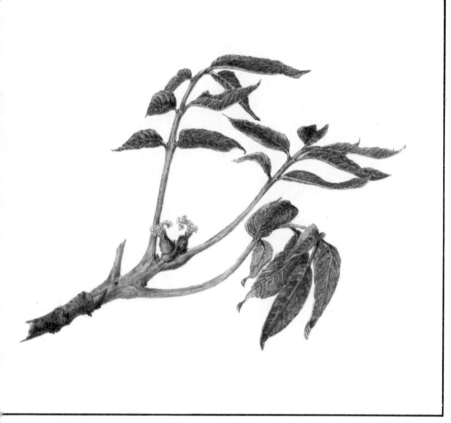

Walnut—Juglans regia

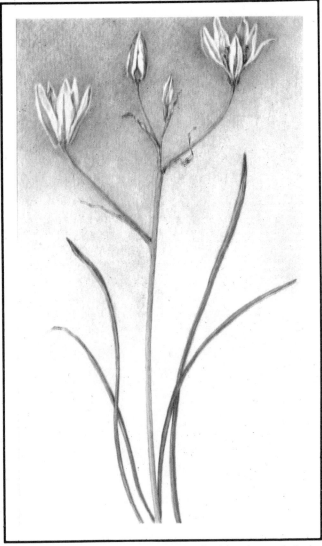

Star of Bethlehem—Ornithogalum umbellatum

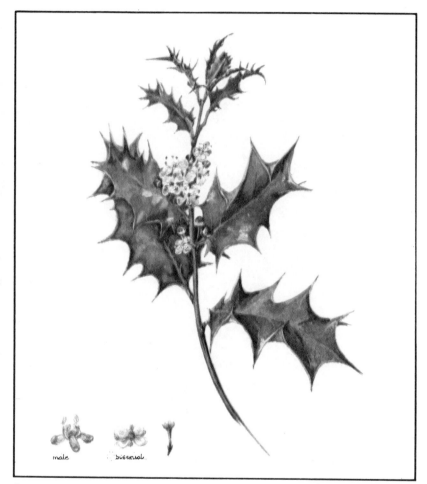

male   bisexual

Holly—Ilex **aquifolium**

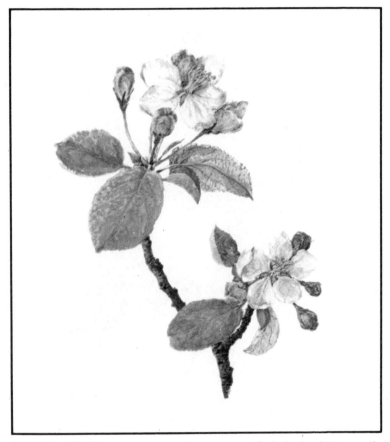

Crab Apple—Malus pumila

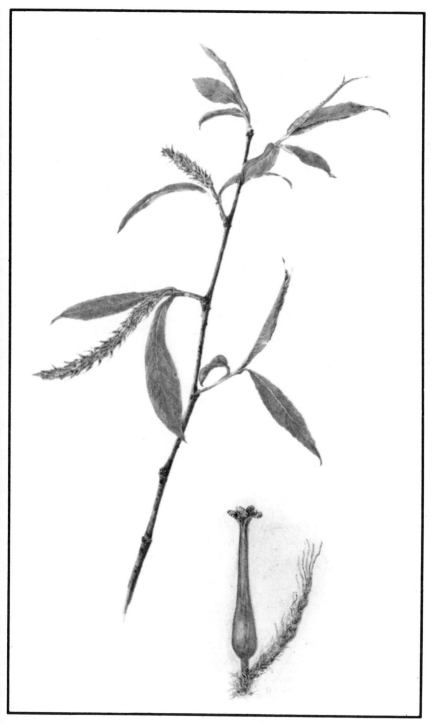

Willow—Salix vitellina

took the Remedies for two days previous to the examinations, and even during them. This time he passed.

Woman, age 76, a widow. She had a bad fall which bruised her face, cut her mouth and twisted her ankle; the injury to the ankle reactivated an old arthritic condition in her back. The accident happened three weeks before she came to us for treatment. When we talked with her, she said that she had lost confidence in her ability to walk safely, and that she could not face the idea of taking a bus, or of even leaving the house. She said: "I am not afraid, but I have lost my confidence, if you can understand the difference." LARCH was given to restore her confidence in herself; STAR OF BETHLEHEM was added to counter any remaining effects of shock. One month later she wrote again to say that she was feeling quite fit again, and that she had fully regained her confidence. What was more, a bronchial condition which she had had for the past year was now completely gone, much to her surprise!

Young man, age 16. He completely lacked confidence in himself. He told us that his father was continually criticizing him, telling him that he was no good, and that he would never "get ahead in life". What was worse, the father often made these discouraging remarks before other people. Consequently, the boy did not try to do anything; not even those things which he could have done easily. He was diffident in the presence of other people, and shy with girls at parties and dances. LARCH was prescribed for his lack of confidence; MIMULUS for his fear and nervousness. The response was immediate, and good. Within the month he wrote to tell us: "The Remedies have worked wonders. I am much more confident, and I am thinking more clearly than before. I enjoy myself at parties and at times I can even come up with a philosophical remark!"

Man, middle age, a vicar. Five years before he came to us, he had a nervous breakdown, and he felt that he had never regained his self-confidence. He continually recalled an incident in his childhood which he said was so vivid in his imagination that it destroyed what little confidence he had left in himself. He suffered from such deep depressions that at times he did not even attempt to preach in his church, and left that duty to the curate. LARCH was given for his lack of self-confidence; HONEYSUCKLE to help him to forget the past; GENTIAN for the depression and discouragement. After three months, he reported that he felt well again, and that he was free from the obsessive incident of his childhood. He resumed his duties toward his church and his congregation, and he did so with enthusiasm and joy.

CHAPTER 21

MIMULUS

Keywords: Fear or anxiety of a *known* origin

THE MIMULUS fear is less acute than the sheer terror of
ROCK ROSE, and it always is caused by known reasons.
Most of us have some pet fear which we would give
much to lose, but which we find hard to overcome at
times. Such fears range from the childhood fear of the
dark, to the fear of growing old, of pain and illness, and
of death itself. These are the MIMULUS fears which
fortunately the Remedy can cure once and for all. The
MIMULUS people are normally shy and retiring; they
are prone to hide their anxieties. They may at times
become tongue-tied with stage fright; again, they can
become garrulous to conceal a nervous fear. They
blush easily, and occasionally they may stammer or
stutter. When they are ill, they are almost afraid to
move lest the pain becomes worse. They sometimes
brood over the possibility of an illness costing them
their job through time lost. During convalescence, they
are afraid to try to exercise an injured limb, or to get
out of bed after an operation; thus they often retard
their own recovery.

The positive aspect of the MIMULUS person is seen in
one who can face all trials and difficulties in life with
equanimity and humor. We fear only those things
which we do not understand, which we dislike, or
which we hate; understanding and courage are the
great positive qualities of the MIMULUS type.

Case Histories

Boy, age 8. He had never been a strong child, and had suffered from birth with an itching eczema around his knees, shortness of breath, and general listlessness. He feared going to the motion pictures, and he disliked having stories read to him lest they turn out badly. He was much too frightened to sleep alone, and seldom slept the night through. MIMULUS the type Remedy was prescribed for his fears and anxieties; CLEMATIS for his dreamy, listless condition. One month later, his mother wrote to say that he was a little better; the eczema was slightly improved, but he still slept badly. The next month she wrote again and said: "Philip is much better in every way. He now sleeps through the night, and is in a room by himself, a thing which he never could do before." Finally, in her last report, three months later, she described her son as being most energetic, without any fears; the eczema had disappeared entirely.

Boy, age 9. His mother wrote: "He is afraid of the teacher at his school, and the work is too difficult for him. He worries about it. He is a very sensitive, kindhearted boy, very sturdy and masculine. This terrible anxiety about school has resulted in his not sleeping well." MIMULUS was prescribed for the boy's fear of his teacher; AGRIMONY for the mental torture and worry about his schoolwork. After the first month, his mother had written to say that the child had lost his fears and was sleeping peacefully again. He had become much more independent, and had said on several occasions: "I can do that for myself." Previously he had been very dependent upon his mother, to whom he was greatly attached.

Boy, age 6. He was very frightened of the dark, and of going up the stairs alone at night. He insisted that a light be always left burning in his room, and that the door remain ajar. During the day he was very energetic, and would not rest; at bedtime he was completely exhausted. His appetite was poor. MIMULUS was prescribed for his fear of the dark; VERVAIN for his excessive energy and his inability to rest. The first report, three weeks later, showed that he was eating better and that he was less exhausted at night. After another two months, his mother wrote to say that he no longer feared the dark; in fact, he even enjoyed switching off the light at bedtime.

Woman, age 29, unmarried. She suffered from arthritis in her left wrist, which had been in a cast for the past two years, and because of that, she had to give up the work she had done on a farm. She was depressed and irritable when she came to us. All her life she had been an unreasonable worrier, nervous, shy, and overconcerned about what other people thought about her. MIMULUS was prescribed for her nervousness, fear and shyness; IMPATIENS for her irritability; GENTIAN for her depression and discouraged attitude. Her first report indicated that there was no change in her wrist, but she said that she was feeling better, and the headache which she usually had during her menstrual period was gone. She had not mentioned the headache during her initial visit, but she was "thrilled" to be without it. The same Remedies were repeated, and four weeks later she wrote to say that she felt like a different person, and the wrist was showing signs of improvement. She said that she had fewer worries and greater happiness than she had had for months. The Remedies were repeated; she again reported an improvement in the wrist, and total absence of headaches during the menstrual period. Her next letter to us related a great setback, and all of her symptoms had returned. The man she had hoped to marry had married another woman. MIMULUS the basic Remedy was prescribed again; STAR OF BETHLEHEM was added for the shock; WILLOW because of the resentment which she bore towards her former fiancé. Within a month, she showed a substantial improvement. Her wrist was still stiff, but not painful. Following this letter, the original prescription was repeated. This resulted in a definite improvement in the wrist, and she herself was much less worried. The same treatment was continued for another three months. She then wrote to say: "The cast has been removed from my wrist. I often forget that there was ever anything wrong with it at all. I am no longer nervous, and I have not had one single headache all of this time. I now no longer worry about what other people say about me."

Boy, age 7. He had just started to go to school, and he was very nervous. He was not sleeping well, and every morning he complained of a pain in his stomach so that he could not eat breakfast. He could not eat his lunch at school, because he was nervous about eating in the presence of strangers. When we saw him, he was pale, listless, and was losing weight. MIMULUS the type Remedy was prescribed, and within a month he was sleeping better. He now not only ate his breakfast, but his lunch at school, and he had gained weight. Most important of all, his mother wrote to say that he liked school and he had said: "I feel as bold as a lion now."

Woman, age 53, married. For many years she had lived in a busy town, and now she found that she could not sleep because of the traffic noise. Noise frightened her, and after working hard all day, she dreaded going home because of it. She was very run down and suffered from morning headaches, as well as a chronic catarrh which blocked her nose. MIMULUS was prescribed for her fear of noise; CRAB APPLE as a cleanser of her system; HORNBEAM to give her strength. After a month, she wrote that she did not feel nearly so tired and that she was sleeping better, but the catarrh persisted. The same Remedies were repeated for another two months. Again she wrote to say that now the fatigue was completely gone, and that she could do twice the amount of work that she normally did; she had lost her fear of noise, and the catarrh had almost cleared up. The next month she wrote again and said that the catarrh had disappeared entirely; she was sleeping well, and she no longer dreaded noise.

Boy, age 13. The boy was a chronic enuretic, and a very heavy sleeper. He was of a cheerful, happy-go-lucky disposition, but his father was a stern disciplinarian and that added to the boy's nervousness. MIMULUS was prescribed for his fear of his father; AGRIMONY for his attitude which concealed his mental torment. During the first three weeks after the treatment started, he wet his bed only once. Four months later, his mother wrote: "A wonderful improvement has taken place. He no longer wets his bed, and he is standing up to his father."

Woman, age 45. She was a business woman whose work entailed standing for long hours, and she suffered from varicose veins. She had lost confidence in herself, and she feared that she might not be able to continue in her business. She wrote to us saying: "I am of a nervous disposition, timid by nature." MIMULUS the type Remedy was prescribed for her nervousness; LARCH for her lack of self-confidence. Her first report was encouraging; she said that she felt much more confidence in herself, and that the veins had improved and the pain stopped. After another four months, she wrote again to say that she felt great confidence in herself and her ability, that she was no longer nervous, and that she was hardly aware of the varicose veins.

CHAPTER 22

MUSTARD

Keywords: Black depression; melancholia; gloom

"THIS Remedy dispels gloom, and brings joy into life" wrote Dr. Bach. The MUSTARD state of mind is a black depression, almost a hopeless, despairing, melancholia which may suddenly close down upon an individual without any apparent reason. It may lift just as suddenly as it comes, but while it lasts, it envelops the person like a black cloud that shuts out all the pleasure and joy of life. The depression is of such a severe nature that it takes away the interest in the daily routine of life. It becomes impossible for the sufferer to be happy, cheerful, or even normal in his thoughts, for they are all turned upon himself. It is all the more distressing because it is impossible to become free of it until it lifts of its own accord, and because there seems to be no explanation for its coming on, or for its leaving. As one patient wrote: "It is as though a cloud descends upon my spirit for no reason. It lasts for a day or two and then it suddenly lifts; it is heavenly to see the light again. I begin to dread this, whatever it is." Another wrote: "I am in a blanket of awful depression with bad headaches. There is nothing I can think of that can cheer me up, nothing seems worthwhile." This state of mind differs from the doubt and discouragement of GENTIAN and from the hopelessness of GORSE because in both of these cases the sufferer knows the cause. The cause of the melancholia of MUSTARD is never known.

The positive aspect of MUSTARD is found in those people who have an inner serenity which nothing can shake or destroy. Such a person is well able to counteract the effect of any attack of melancholia or depression by his inner stability, joy and peace.

CASE HISTORIES

Woman, age 50, married. She lived in a beautiful house, and she had two grown sons, both of whom were very successful men. At times, throughout her life, she suffered from acute attacks of depression for no known reason. The attack would come on suddenly without any warning; it would continue for some days, and then it would disappear as suddenly as it came. While the depression lasted, it seemed like a long black night to her. She lost interest in everything, and she could see nothing beautiful or bright around her. She longed to overcome these depressions, because she had so many things to do, and she felt rather ashamed that she could not overcome them. MUSTARD the type Remedy was prescribed. During the first two months, she had but one attack, and that lasted one day only. She continued to take the Remedy for several months more, as she said: "Just to be sure that I am strong enough to rise above this depression." She has not reported having had any more attacks.

Woman, middle age, unmarried. She worked in a busy hospital, but she was forced to resign because she suffered such severe depressions that she was unable to continue her work. At first she thought that she was overtired, but she liked her work, and that did not seem to be the cause; there was no apparent reason for the depressions. The rest that she thought would help her only increased the depression and caused anxiety about her financial situation. She told us that she was never aggressive by nature, and that this had hindered her progress through life. She said that people tended to avoid her, and she had few friends. She was beginning to feel hopeless about herself. MUSTARD was prescribed for her black depression; GORSE for her hopeless outlook. Her report, one month later, was encouraging. She said: "I am feeling much better. My problems are far from solved, but I do feel more able to face them instead of allowing them to overwhelm me." Two months later, she wrote again to say that the depressions had disappeared and she was so much happier. She was making plans for the future, and her life was very much brighter.

Man, middle age, who held a very important post in Nigeria wrote to us to say that he was losing interest in his work, and that he was mentally and physically exhausted. His physicians were greatly puzzled, and though he was not anemic, they nevertheless suspected pernicious anemia. Throughout his life he had suffered from periods of black depressions without apparent cause. The following prescription was sent to him by mail: MUSTARD the type Remedy for the black depressions; OLIVE for his mental and physical exhaustion. Two months later he wrote to say that he felt in far better shape than he had for a long time previously; we quote from his letter: "I am reluctantly obliged to attribute the improvement to the Bach Remedies as I refuse to have blind faith in something I know nothing about." The same Remedies were repeated, and three months later he wrote again to say that he was in excellent health, and his depressions had gone. Two years later he wrote again to say: "I am very well, thanks to the Bach Remedies. The depressions have never recurred."

Woman, age 21, unmarried. She was subject to attacks of black depressions for which there was no known cause. She had always been inclined to be pessimistic. She found it difficult to make friends, and she felt cut off from the company of other people. MUSTARD was prescribed as the type Remedy for her deep melancholia. After two months, she wrote to say that she felt as if a cloud had lifted from her mind, and that she really was happy. Later, her mother wrote to say that she had become an altogether different person. She was now taking part in many activities, and she had made many new friends.

Woman, age 39, married. She suffered from severe depressions and she felt as if a black cloud enveloped her which shut her off from the rest of the world. She could not think of any reason for the depressions. She could only say that they came on suddenly, and that she was helpless to do anything about them until they passed of their own accord. When she came to us, she was a very unhappy and depressed person. She was also suffering from an acute cystitis which seemed to be getting worse, and from constipation. She said that she was a nervously tense person, and that she could never relax. MUSTARD was prescribed for the deep depressions; VERVAIN for her inability to relax. The first improvement was physical; both the cystitis and the constipation improved. She continued to take the medicine for several weeks more; after a period of five weeks she said that she had not had any more attacks of depression and that she felt better in every way. Shortly thereafter she suffered a setback. She had a boil in her ear, and that brought back the depressions again. CRAB APPLE to cleanse her system, together with GENTIAN for discouragement were added to the basic prescription. The next month she wrote to say that the boil had burst the second day, and had given no more trouble, but most important of all, the depressions had gone; she said she was feeling happy and on top of the world. So far as is known, the depressions have never returned.

Woman, age 67, a widow. She told us that from time to time, even as a child, her life had been a black misery. Periods of deep depression had filled her with despair, and she said: "Why they come, I do not know." During the attacks her head throbbed; she slept badly because of recurring nightmares which wakened her. She was taking sleeping tablets, but they did not seem to help her much. MUSTARD was prescribed for the dark depressions and melancholia; ROCK ROSE for the terror of the nightmares. Her response was very rapid. She said that after the first week she was able to give up the sleeping tablets, and that although she still had nightmares, they were vague and ill-defined, and did not trouble her. After another two months, she was able to write:

"My mind is at rest after so many years of anguish. I am no longer the victim of those black depressions." Six months later she wrote again to say that she was well and happy, and that the melancholia had never returned.

Woman, age 45, married. She suffered greatly from deep melancholia which came upon her without warning, and for no known reason. During the attacks, she felt utterly alone, and that nothing could ever help her. When she sought our help, she was suffering from acute lumbago, and was confined to bed. This fact increased her nervous tension, because it was essential that she return to work as soon as possible. MUSTARD was prescribed for the black depressions; IMPATIENS for the tension which caused the pain; GORSE for her feeling of hopelessness. The next week she wrote to say: "The medicine is really doing me good. My back is well again, and I am able to go back to work." After another two months of treatment, she wrote again saying: "I feel better than I have felt for years. I have no more depressions or moments of hopelessness. If either ever should occur, I will write to you again." We have never heard from her since.

CHAPTER 23

OAK

Keywords: Despondency; despair; but never-ceasing effort

THE OAK people struggle on in the face of every difficulty. They never give up hope. They are ceaseless in
their efforts to find a cure when they are sick; they are
untiring in their efforts to improve their condition.
They are the exact opposite of the GORSE type who are
ready to give up trying when things look hopeless.
Though the OAK type may feel despondent, and though
they may often suffer from despair due to the conditions imposed upon them, they will continue to fight.
If their poor health interferes with their work, they
become disappointed and discontented with themselves. They are reliable, dependable people, so much
so that others tend to lay their burdens on their
shoulders, and to pass their responsibilities to them.
The OAK type likes to help other people of their own
free will, and for this reason, they sometimes overwork.
They are the mainstay of the family, and sometimes
they plod on from day to day, hiding their tiredness
or ill health from others lest their despair or despondency be discovered. The OAK type, like the tree itself,
are strong physically, and they can stand great strain;
they are very patient, and full of common sense. Yet
there can come a time when the despondency and
the despair becomes too much for human endurance;
then it is when the OAK person can crack, and suffer
a nervous breakdown.

Dr. Bach described the positive aspects of the OAK type in these words: "They are brave people, fighting against great difficulties without loss of hope or slackening of effort." They reflect perseverence, courage and stability under all conditions.

CASE HISTORIES

Woman, age 42, unmarried. She held a responsible and busy job, and had a home to look after as well. When she came to see us, she said that she was tired to the point of exhaustion but went on in spite of that. She was discontented with herself; every month she suffered from such a severe migraine headache that she had to stay home from work. She was a very conscientious and reserved person. She was suffering from insomnia, and occasional periods of despondency. OAK the type Remedy was prescribed for her conscientiousness, her sense of responsibility, and her hidden despondency; OLIVE for the exhaustion of mind and body. The first report was encouraging. She had an attack of migraine, but she could nevertheless go to work that day; she felt less tired, and she was sleeping better. She continued to take the same Remedies, and the next month she said that apart from a minor headache, she was feeling much better. Two months later she wrote that she had never felt better in her whole life, and that she had no more headaches. She was now able to assume all of her many responsibilities once more.

Woman, middle age, unmarried. She was the headmistress of an infants' school. When she came to see us, she said that she felt her responsibilities were becoming too much for her, although she would never admit that to others. She suffered from stress and consequent indigestion. The parents, as well as the children, constantly came to her for advice because of her stable character and practical common sense. OAK was prescribed for her struggle against tiredness in her work; GENTIAN from the resulting depression. Within three months she reported good progress in every way. She was no longer fatigued, and was not troubled with indigestion. She said that she was well able to cope with both children and parents, as well as all of the work connected with the school. She continued to take the Remedies for another month, and felt completely cured.

Man, age 45. He came to see us during the war. Before the war started, he had been afflicted with asthma, and now he had had an attack of pleurisy. He had been given one month's leave of absence from work, but instead of taking the full time, he had returned to work too soon. He was on the night shift, and said, simply: "It was my job, my war-effort, so I had to stick to it." He was then given a clerical job, under two bosses. These people gave conflicting orders, but once again, though this caused him confusion and distress, he simply said: "I had to stick it." The stress engendered brought on a severe attack of asthma, which was followed by other attacks of increasing severity. Though he was of a nervous disposition, and lacking in self-confidence, he concealed the fact well, and he struggled on with his work. OAK was prescribed for his valiant efforts to keep working; MIMULUS for his nervousness; LARCH for his lack of confidence in himself. After the first month, he reported that he felt better in every way; things were running more smoothly for him, and he felt more confident. After another two months, he was able to breathe normally again; the asthma had completely disappeared. He was feeling well, and regarded his work with pleasure. He suffered no relapse.

Man, age 38, a schoolmaster by profession. Fifteen years before he came to us, he had suffered a nervous breakdown, and for two years afterwards, he was unable to work. Finally he recovered enough to teach again, although he still lacked confidence in himself. Now he held a position of responsibility at the school. He struggled on courageously, hiding his fatigue and his depressions because he wanted nothing to interfere with his work. OAK was prescribed for his courageous struggle; HORNBEAM to give him mental and physical strength; MIMULUS for the occasional fear that he might give in. He continued the treatment for three months, and as a result he became more confident, more at peace, and happier. He wrote to us saying: "There is a subtle difference in me which I am unable to explain, but all is going well with me now."

Woman, middle age, a widow. She had one grown son whom she had succeeded in putting through school in spite of her own poor health. She had never thought of giving up the struggle, and now she was very proud of this boy who had a good job in the United States. At the time that she came to us for treatment, she was suffering from leukorrhea, and passing through the climacteric. She was indeed a brave woman, one who always appeared to be self-possessed. But in spite of her outwardly calm appearance, she was depressed by her many difficulties. OAK the type Remedy was prescribed for her valiant struggle against great odds; CRAB APPLE as a cleansing Remedy; GENTIAN for the depression which she concealed so successfully. She responded quickly to the treatment and after a month she wrote: "My general health has greatly improved. The leukorrhea has cleared up entirely, and for almost the first time in my life, I am feeling on tip-toe."

Man, age 48. He was a business man, and very occupied with several companies, family worries, and other responsibilities. Outwardly he was placid, but for some years he had suffered from sinus trouble, and catarrh of the nose and throat. This condition was so severe that he had to use an inhaler continually, especially at night, otherwise he was unable to breathe through his nose. In spite of these difficulties, he never missed a day from his work, and fought all of the time to keep going. He had tried many treatments at the hands of different specialists, but every winter the condition returned, and he was fast becoming despondent at the thought of ever being cured. OAK the type Remedy was prescribed for his courageous efforts to keep going; CRAB APPLE as a cleanser; HORNBEAM to give him strength and vitality. After the first month of treatment, he was able to dispense with the inhaler entirely, and to breathe through his nose, even at night. After another month, he wrote to say that he was enjoying the best winter season for many years; he was without sinus trouble, and the catarrh had almost cleared up. One month later he wrote again to say that he was feeling fine. The catarrh had disappeared entirely, and he could report no trouble at all. After many years, he wrote again to say that none of his symptoms had recurred.

Woman, age 40, single. Her health had been poor during her entire life. When she came to us for treatment, she was suffering from hay-fever and hemorrhoids. She told us that she was accident-prone, and that some years before she had fallen and injured her spine, with the result that she had to be several months in a hospital. She was told that she would eventually be unable to walk, and that with time she would become paralysed. In spite of this dire prognosis, she said: "I refused to believe it. I had to earn my living, so I had to work." Now she is even walking a long distance to her work every day! She then said that she found it difficult to relax, and that she often woke in the morning with her teeth and hands clenched tightly. OAK the type Remedy was prescribed for her valiant struggle; VERVAIN for the tension of mind and body; HONEYSUCKLE to remove, once and for all, the unfortunate threat that she might become paralysed. Within two months time, she was a different person. The hay-fever had disappeared. The hemorrhoids had receded and were normal. She slept well, and woke refreshed and relaxed. She was able to say: "For the first time in my life I feel really well."

CHAPTER 24

OLIVE

Keywords: Complete exhaustion; mental fatigue

THE Olive tree benefits humanity through its leaves, bark, fruit, and the wood of its trunk. It has always been the symbol of peace and harmony. The Remedy prepared from the Olive flowers has the power to restore peace to the tired mind, and strength to a body exhausted by suffering. It is the Remedy for those persons who have suffered a long time under adverse conditions, or who have had a long and grievous illness which has sapped their vitality; their minds have become wearied and exhausted, and their reserve strength is depleted. As one patient said: "I am suffering from utter weariness and a complete lack of zest." Another: "I am exhausted to the point of tears." OLIVE also helps those persons who live full lives, and have very much to do, so much so that they have little time for leisure and relaxation. They tire easily and quickly, and they have no reserve of strength to carry on with. Everything has become an effort for them, and, because they are so tired, they no longer enjoy their work, or those things which once gave them pleasure or interest. The OLIVE exhaustion is different from that of HORNBEAM. The latter is a fatigue of the mind, and a disinclination to face the future or even daily routine; yet as the day progresses, the sufferer finds that he can indeed fulfil his appointed tasks. The fatigue of the OLIVE type is total; mind and body are drained of strength, and there is absolute exhaustion. OLIVE is also the Remedy to give during convalescence from a long illness. It restores vitality, strength, and indeed, an interest in life itself.

The positive aspects of the OLIVE folk is seen in those people who do not rely upon personal effort to over-come their difficulties. They rely instead upon that strength and vitality which they know will be given to them and which will sustain them and guide them in every respect. It is seen in those who maintain their peace of mind and their interest in life, even though they may be forced to remain inactive. Of the OLIVE type, in their positive aspects, it might be said: "They also serve who only stand and wait."

CASE HISTORIES

Woman, age 64, married. Within the last few years, all her family, those close to her, her husband, her child and her brother had died. Since that time she had felt completely exhausted and life seemed to hold little for her. She said: "I am not particularly interested in anything, and I do not have the energy to do anything about it." She was depressed, and she slept badly. OLIVE was prescribed for her utter exhaus-tion, her loss of interest and her depression. She took this regularly for three months; she was soon able to report that she was sleeping better, and for longer hours, and that she was eating again, and gaining weight. At the end of four months she wrote to say: "I am much better, and I am getting about once again. I sleep wonderfully well. The depressions are things of the past."

Woman, age 50, a widow. She was the mother of two grown sons, for whom she kept house. The house was large, and the work overtaxed her strength. She became very tired, and suffered from severe depressions. She told us that she had never fully recovered from a hysterectomy the year before. OLIVE was prescribed for her state of exhaustion; MUSTARD for the severe black depressions. After three months, she wrote to say that she was feeling much better and that she was well able to cope with all of her household duties without getting overtired. Most important of all, she had not had any depressions for the last six weeks.

Woman, age 73, a widow. She had recently been under a strain due to family difficulties. She said to us: "I suddenly get exhausted, as if I had nothing at all inside of me." The years of worry had left her feeling weak, and unable to cope with the problems life posed. OLIVE was prescribed, and she took this for a long while. Gradually her strength returned, and she was once again able to face the problems that confronted her.

Woman, age 60, a widow. She was an active and intense person by nature, and inclined to overtax her strength. For the last three years, she looked after her daughter's baby, while the daughter was at work, and this had brought her to the point of exhaustion. Her life had been a difficult one. Her husband had died after a lingering illness, and she had to earn her own living to support her child. When she came to us, she was near complete exhaustion, and she had been spitting blood for some months. She was resentful of many things, although, as she admitted, she had no reason to be. OLIVE was prescribed for her exhausted condition; WILLOW for her resentment; CRAB APPLE to cleanse her system from the toxins of fatigue. After taking the Remedies for one month, she reported that she no longer spat blood, and although she was still tired, she was much less resentful. She continued to take the Remedies for another two months. Once during this period she had a return of the bloody sputum, but only for a short while. She said that she had recovered her full strength again, and that she was once more a cheerful, happy person.

Woman, age 73, married. By nature, she was a kind and gentle person, much giving to daydreaming. For the last three months, she had been extremely busy and overworked. Suddenly she found that her right hand could not hold a pen or a teacup; when she tried to write, the letters were all jumbled together. She had taken to her bed in a state of complete exhaustion, and had apparently lost interest in everything. OLIVE was prescribed for the exhaustion; CLEMATIS for the tendency to daydream. Her reaction was quick and certain. After taking the Remedies for two months, she reported that she felt like her old self again, and that her strength and interest in life had returned.

Woman, age 39, unmarried. She held the post of Occupational Therapy Officer in a large town, and she was greatly overworked. One day she suffered a blackout and was confined to a nursing home for a month. When she came to us for treatment, she was still weak, and had lost interest in her work. To make matters worse, she had been told that the blackout could be caused by epilepsy, or by a brain tumor, and this caused her great concern and mental anguish. In the nursing home, she had been given large doses of phenobarbital, and when she was discharged she was still too weak to return to work. OLIVE was prescribed for her exhaustion; HONEYSUCKLE to help her forget the frightening diagnosis. She recovered rapidly, and within three months she was well and back at work. She wrote: "I really do feel lots better, and I have regained my strength again. I can hardly believe it!"

Woman, middle age, a widow. Her husband was killed in the crash of a commercial airliner two years before. She had heard the first report about the accident over the radio, and naturally the shock was very great. Since then she had lost interest in life and seemed unable to make any effort to recover from the extreme fatigue from which she was suffering. Her thoughts were continually on the past. She suffered from many physical ailments, and felt that life held nothing for her any longer. OLIVE was prescribed for her mental and physical exhaustion; WHITE CHESTNUT to clear her mind of the recurring thoughts; STAR OF BETHLEHEM to counteract the shock. She responded well to the Remedies. Within two months she was able to report that she had gained her peace of mind again. Her strength had returned, she was taking a lively interest in things, and had in fact resumed most of her former activities.

Woman, age 46, unmarried. During the past years, she had many illnesses. She was unhappy in her work because she had too much to do. Her mother was an invalid, and she was the sole support of her younger sister. When she came to us for treatment, she was about at the end of her rope. She was suffering from palpitations, she saw spots before her eyes, and her ears rang continually. She was so exhausted in body and mind that she felt she could not carry on another minute. OLIVE was prescribed for the extreme exhaustion. She took the Remedy for two months. Her strength returned; the palpitations, the spots before the eyes, and the ringing in her ears had disappeared. She was once again able to do her work without undue fatigue, and she could stand up against an abusive employer.

CHAPTER 25

PINE

Keywords: Self-reproach; guilt feelings; despondency

PINE is the Remedy for those people who suffer from self-condemnation, who are never really content with their achievements, and who blame themselves for not doing better. They also tend to blame themselves for the mistakes of others, for they feel that in some way they themselves are responsible. A typical PINE statement is: "I am always tired and depressed, and feel that I am the worst person in the world. I blame myself for everything that goes wrong in the house." They are overconcientious, and the high standards they set themselves (although not for others) may cause them to overwork and bring about emotional stress in their effort to "improve" their characters. When they become ill, they blame themselves for their failure towards their family, their friends, or their work. The guilt-complex from which they suffer takes much of the joy out of their lives. As one said: "I feel so guilty accepting this extra money although I do need it so badly. There are many other people much worse off than I." Another said: "As you know, I have had no home for a long time and I have just seen a little apartment which would be perfect for me. But I do feel that if I take it I shall blame myself for doing so, when there are so many others who are in need of a home." The PINE type are the opposite of the WILLOW people, for the latter put the blame for their mistakes on others, and they become resentful and bitter towards them. The PINE type also differ from the ROCK WATER persons, for the ROCK WATER persons are hard masters on themselves from a sense of spiritual pride; they suppress their faults, and enjoy doing so. Though the PINE type are too humble and apologetic, they do things well, and actually have every reason to be content with their capabilities. They are unlike the LARCH type who will not try because they fear failure; the PINE type will put his hand to anything, and will try his best to do well. But when he cannot live up to the high ideal he has set for himself, he becomes depressed and even despondent, and he may well sink into listless despair. All of these four types, PINE, WILLOW, ROCK WATER and LARCH are a group. Of them, Dr. Bach wrote: "[They have not yet come to realize] one trace of condemnation against ourselves, or others, is a trace of condemnation against the Universal Creation of Love, and restricts us, limits our power to allow the Universal Love to flow through us to others."* Also, as Dr. Bach wrote elsewhere: "No great ascent was ever made without faults and falls, and they must be regarded as experiences which will help us to stumble less in the future. No thoughts of past errors must ever depress us; they are over and finished and the knowledge thus gained will help us to avoid a repetition of them."

The positive aspects of the PINE type is seen in those people who are willing to take the responsibility and to bear the burdens of others if they can really help them. They are aware, however, that this is not always the best way to help another. The PINE persons acknowledge their mistakes, but do not dwell upon them; they

---

* *Heal Thyself* by Edward Bach. The C. W. Daniel Company Ltd., Ashingdon, Rochford, Essex, England; 9th edition 1970.

have great perseverence, and a genuine humility about their talents.

Case Histories

Woman, age 45, unmarried. During an interview she said: "I am always blaming myself for not having done something I feel that I ought to have done, or now, because I am ill and I have to stay away from work and others will have more to do. I feel terribly ashamed, and have a sense of guilt. I have sagging internal organs and much discomfort; also I am tired and feel that I shall never be well again." PINE was prescribed for the sense of guilt and self-condemnation; GORSE for the hopelessness. She took these for one month, and at the next interview she said: "I am very much better in many ways, but I am still inclined to feel guilty, and I feel that I ought to return to work although I am still very tired, and I have little interest in things". OLIVE was added to the prescription for her fatigue, and the results were good. After another month she said: "I have more vitality and strength, but I have overdone things, and that put me back. But, strangely enough, I am not blaming myself for that!" The Remedies were repeated for another three months. She said in her last interview, that she had had no more discomfort in her abdomen for several months, and "I see how foolish it is to keep blaming myself for so many things; I am learning the lesson, thanks to you."

Woman, middle age, widowed. She had a grown son who lived with her. Recently she had begun to blame herself for not being able to make him happy in his home because he thought of going to the United States to seek work. She was suffering from leukorrhea and that made her feel unclean. PINE was prescribed for her sense of guilt; CRAB APPLE to cleanse her mind and body. At the end of the first month she wrote: "I have derived great benefit. The leukorrhea has now disappeared and I am feeling really well again. I feel happy for my son who went to the United States and has been doing well there."

Woman, age 65, married. She had suffered from acute sciatica for the past six months. The pain was so severe that at times she would scream. She had tried several treatments, but mostly without success. By nature, she was shy and diffident. She was overwhelmed with the idea of guilt, and she was certain that she was being punished, and that she deserved to be. She recently had a great shock when a friend of hers died during the night, and she was not aware of it until the morning when she found her body. PINE the type Remedy was prescribed for the feeling of guilt; STAR OF BETHLEHEM for the shock her friend's death occasioned; MIMULUS for her diffidence and shyness. After the first three weeks, she felt greatly improved, although she still had a pain in her left leg. The same Remedies were repeated, and the next month she reported: "I see now that I could not have saved my friend, and I do not blame myself any more. The pain has all cleared wonderfully; it has just gone away."

Man, age 59, a dental surgeon by profession, in private practice. He was by nature a calm and painstaking man who would do almost anything to avoid a disagreement. He worried unduly about things he could do quite well, and his life was a continual stress. His wife had nine nervous breakdowns since their marriage many years before, and he blamed himself for these. He worked hard at his practice, and also did the housework and tended the garden when his wife was indisposed. When he talked with us, he said that his chief concern was that he could not do more for his wife. He felt frustrated. He was fatigued and held himself responsible for anything that went wrong. He suffered from a high index of uric acid in his blood and he was subject to acute attacks of gout. PINE was prescribed for his self accusations; CRAB APPLE to cleanse his system of the excess uric acid; AGRIMONY as his type Remedy. After about six weeks, he reported that the gout had almost disappeared and that he could work in the garden again, and also he was sleeping better than he had been able to do for years. The next month he wrote again to report a setback. He had been under a terrible strain; one of his daughters had married, and his wife had another break-

down. The gout had returned, but it was milder than usual.
PINE was prescribed again; ELM for his many responsibilities;
CRAB APPLE and AGRIMONY. The gout cleared up quickly.
He said that he could cope with his responsibilities once more.
After another month, he wrote: "I have really been benefited.
I do not reproach myself, or worry about my wife any more.
It seems strange not to worry like that after all of these years.
I now take things easier, and the general condition of my
health is excellent."

Woman, age 58, unmarried. She was the secretary to an
important health organization. When she came to us, she was
completely exhausted from overwork, and on the verge of a
nervous breakdown. Interviewing patients and answering the
telephone all day seemed beyond her capabilities. She suffered from palpitations, weakness of the knees, cold shivers
and insomnia. Her chief concern was that she was letting
down her employer with whom she had worked for many
years. She blamed herself for not feeling well, and for not
being able to do her work as usual. PINE was prescribed for
her self-blame; OLIVE for exhaustion, and she was advised to
take a long vacation to regain her strength. At first she
refused even to consider this, because the Remedies had
given her strength. Finally she realized that in spite of that,
she must rest because she was still weak, and not able to work
at full capacity. She retired from work and went to live by
the sea. She regained her health completely and has been well
since that time. Now she is over seventy and is the picture of
good health and happy spirits.

Woman, age 50, unmarried. In her interview with us she
said: "I have a great sense of guilt and shame for no reason;
it makes me most unhappy. I have sagging abdominal organs,
and although I am under the care of an osteopathic physician,
I feel that I shall never really improve." PINE the type Remedy
was prescribed for her sense of self-condemnation; GENTIAN
for her doubt that she would get better. The response was
rapid, and she felt so well that she overtaxed her strength and
suffered a setback. HORNBEAM was added to give her strength.
After another two months, she was able to report that she had

no further abdominal discomfort, nor was she reproachful of herself. Much later she wrote to say that she had had no recurrence of her physical or emotional difficulties.

Woman, young, married. She had adopted twin boys, four years old. They were lively youngsters, always on the go, and she found it exhausting to keep up with them all day long; nevertheless she tried to, because she loved them dearly. She reproached herself severely and blamed herself for becoming impatient and irritated with them. Because of constant tension she could not sleep at night, and was exhausted during the day. She had developed a mastitis in her left breast which troubled her greatly. PINE was prescribed for her self-reproach; IMPATIENS for her impatience and irritability. She took the Remedies for one month, and was able to report excellent results. The mastitis was completely cured; she no longer blamed herself, and she did not become impatient or irritated with the twins.

CHAPTER 26

RED CHESTNUT

Keywords: Excessive fear; anxiety for others

DR. BACH described the Remedy thus: "The RED CHESTNUT fear is for others, especially those dear to us. If they return home late, there is the thought that some accident may have happened; if they go for a holiday, there is the dread that some calamity will befall them. There is great anxiety for those who are not even dangerously ill, and a minor ailment becomes a major complaint in the imagination. It is always fearing the worst, and always anticipating misfortune for others." This is also the fear which causes a contraction of breath when we see a child crossing the road in front of an oncoming automobile, or someone slipping from an unsteady ladder. A few days before he discovered RED CHESTNUT, Dr. Bach had a bad accident with an axe; this caused great anxiety on the part of those close to him as immediate first aid was applied to stanch the blood. When he had recovered, Dr. Bach said that we had experienced the state of mind of the next Remedy which he would seek; a Remedy to counteract the fear for others. He also added that our anxiety on his behalf, although we had done our best to hide it, had not helped him at all. His sensitivity was so great that he could not avoid sensing and reacting to our feelings of the moment; any thought of depression, worry or fear in another person would cause him acute physical pain. Let us never forget that negative thoughts not only harm us, but also those around us!

The positive aspect of this Remedy is the ability to send out thoughts of safety, health or courage to those who need them, and who may be in danger or ill at the time. It is the ability to remain calm, mentally and physically, in any emergency.

CASE HISTORIES

Man, age 60. When he applied to us for treatment, he was suffering from a bad skin eruption on his feet which affected both the plantar and dorsal surfaces. Blisters formed, burst, and the skin became hard and scaly, with intense irritation. The process repeated its cycle continually, and had done so since it first appeared some eighteen years before. At that time, his son had an accident. He fractured his arm and it later became paralysed. It was a great shock to the father, and caused him great anxiety. A few days later the skin condition became manifest. After an X-ray treatment, it disappeared for a while, but ten years later, when he broke two bones in his foot, it reappeared. Again it was treated by X-rays and again it disappeared only to appear some years later when he broke his femur; the same sequence once more: X-ray, disappearance. The next year he was operated on to remove his right kidney. The operation was most successful, but the rash reappeared, and the roentgenologist refused to give him any more X-ray treatments because of possible over-exposure. He was given lotions and salves, but they did not help. We found him in a very poor condition of health; his feet were inflamed, and the irritation was intense, so intense that he could not sleep. He was very fatigued, nervous, and had lost his appetite. He said that he was beginning to shun people and to lose interest in life. He said: "It seems ages since life held any sparkle for me." But what worried him the most was the possibility of losing his job and not being able to support his family. He could imagine them in his mind's eye, homeless and starving. RED CHESTNUT was prescribed for his anxiety over his family; STAR OF BETHLEHEM for the shocks he had experienced; CRAB APPLE to cleanse mind and body. Within a month, he reported that the irritation on his feet was less, and the inflammation reduced. He felt that his general health had improved, and he was able to get a good night's sleep. The same Remedies were repeated, and four months after, he reported that his general health was very good, and the skin condition had once again disappeared. He wrote: "Since taking the Remedies my outlook on life has changed, and very much too! I am most grateful."

Woman, age 38, married. Her husband was ill with a nervous breakdown, and her six-year-old son was diabetic. As she said to us: "I really have been ill and exhausted for a year, and the other day I lost all feeling in my right leg, from the hip to the ankle. I am always worried about my husband and my son. If they are out of sight I am anxious in case something might happen to them. Every morning when I awake, I wonder whether my son is worse." RED CHESTNUT was prescribed for her abnormal anxiety over her husband and her son; VERVAIN for the tension and stress. She took these Remedies for two months. Shortly after she started to take them, the feeling returned to her leg; she grew much calmer, and she was able to sleep well again. Although her husband had to be confined in hospital, she said that she felt much less worried about him than she did before. She felt stronger, and she said that she was very hopeful about the future. She was even considering adopting another little boy as a companion for her son.

Woman, elderly, a grandmother. She had cared for her grandson ever since his mother's death, and she took her responsibility very seriously. She was over-anxious about him, wondering whether he would meet with an accident on the way to school, or whether he would catch cold in the rain. She was filled with fear about him all of the time. She herself suffered from frequent colds, indigestion, and persistent headaches. RED CHESTNUT the type Remedy was prescribed for her over-concern for the grandchild; WHITE CHESTNUT because she was continually thinking about his safety and well-being. Within one week after taking the Remedies she said that she felt better than she had for a long while. She continued to take the Remedies for another six weeks. At the end of that time, she was free of colds and the digestive disturbances. She said that she felt happier, and much less worried about her grandson; she even said that he seemed quite capable of taking care of himself.

Woman, elderly, married. Her husband had just suffered a heart attack. She herself was quite frail, and distressed and concerned about his condition. RED CHESTNUT was prescribed for her concern about her husband; CHERRY PLUM because it was feared that her mind was strained to the point where she could have a nervous breakdown. She continued to nurse her husband while she took the Remedies. After the first month, her daughter wrote to say that she was amazed to see how well her mother was now, and that she never would have thought that such a change was possible in so short a time.

Woman, middle age, a widow. Her daughter had idealized her father, and when he died she blamed her mother for his death. The daughter had just had a miscarriage, and this added stress to the psychological barrier which already existed between the two women. The mother had been, by nature, a happy and cheerful woman; a practical kind of person, with many interests. When she came to us for treatment, the tension between her daughter and herself had taken its toll; she was suffering from poor circulation, constipation, and insomnia. RED CHESTNUT was prescribed because of her concern about her daughter's health and attitude; CRAB APPLE as a cleanser of mind and body; VERVAIN for the tension that had arisen between the two persons. Within two weeks, she reported that she was feeling much better. The tension had lessened markedly, and the constipation was beginning to respond to the treatment. She took the medicine for another six weeks, when she was able to report: "The constipation has almost become a thing of the past. I am enjoying life once more, and I do not feel any anxiety about my daughter now.

We are good friends again, and I am sure that is because of my changed attitude towards her."

Woman, age 75, a widow. She wrote to us as follows: "Since I have been taking the Remedy (RED CHESTNUT) which you sent to me, my health is much better, and the difference I will try to explain. I have always been keenly concerned about my daughter's ups and downs, eager to help her when necessary, and worried when I could not do so. Now I do not seem to worry so much, and although I live quite near her, I only go to see her when she says she needs me. I am no longer always worrying about what she is doing, or whether or not she is able to manage things. The medicine you sent me has brought about this happy condition, and I am most grateful."

Woman, age 70, married. Her 80-year-old husband was in a hospital waiting to undergo a serious operation. She was very concerned about him, and anxious about his chances of surviving the operation. She stayed awake at night worrying about him, and she forgot or neglected to prepare herself proper meals. RED CHESTNUT alone was prescribed. After a few weeks she could sleep well again, and she regained her appetite. She saw her husband every day, and she said that she was able to talk with him in a bright and cheerful manner. She herself felt optimistic and very well.

CHAPTER 27

ROCK ROSE

Keywords: Terror; panic; extreme fright

ROCK ROSE is the Remedy to be given whenever terror is experienced, whether the person is in good health or not. People who are suffering from this state of mind are usually in a serious condition; the Remedy is needed on such occasions, or when there has been an accident or near-escape. *It is also useful when the situation of the patient is so grave that it affects those around him.* In other words, give ROCK ROSE whenever there is terror in the atmosphere, both to the patient and to those near to him. One patient, who recovered from an illness remarked concerning the attitude of those around him: "They tell me I was unconscious; anyway, I was so peaceful and comfortable. Then something hit me like a blow; it hurt, and I felt pain, and I was so ill. I tried to push it away, whatever it was. I learned later that at just that time, my wife and daughter had been told to expect the worst." Extreme fear or terror may assail those facing an unexpected or unfamiliar experience. It is also induced by a terrifying sight such as the bodies of victims in an accident; fortunately, it is only a temporary state of mind. Children often experience terror after a nightmare; whenever great fear is experienced, four drops of ROCK ROSE in a little water should be sipped at frequent intervals; it will quickly sooth and calm the sufferer.

The positive aspects of ROCK ROSE are seen in military

or civil heroes, those courageous persons who are willing to risk their lives to aid others. It is a state of mind wherein the self is completely forgotten.

CASE HISTORIES

Girl, age 12. A tragedy happened to one of her schoolmates and this terrified her. She began to have nightmares that caused her to cry out, to toss and turn all night long, and to walk in her sleep. She was by nature a high-strung child, and the terror caused her to lose her appetite. She was losing weight rapidly. ROCK ROSE the type Remedy was prescribed for her terror. After the first two days, she stopped walking in her sleep, but she was still restless, disturbed, and talked in her sleep. By the end of the first month, she was sleeping peacefully and was calmer, happier, and was eating again. HONEYSUCKLE was added to ROCK ROSE to help her forget the events of the past. After five months, her mother wrote to say that she had completely recovered, that she was now well, and emotionally stable.

Man, middle age. He was a patient in a hospital where he was critically ill with a paralysed intestine following a major abdominal operation. Because of his great fear, which the panic and terror of his wife amplified, he was given a sip of ROCK ROSE every ten minutes. Half an hour after the first dose, peristaltic action was restored, and he had a bowel movement. This saved his life. Subsequently he was given other Remedies in conformation with his moods until he had completely recovered.

Woman, age 54, a widow. She was terrified by all forms of travel: bus, train or car. She could never sleep the night before she had to undertake a journey, and she felt that literally she "fell to pieces" from panic. On such occasions, she suffered severe headaches, and her hands trembled so much that she was unable to button her coat, or to hold her handbag. ROCK ROSE the type Remedy was prescribed, and she was advised to take an extra dose just before she had to travel. After one month she wrote to us to say: "I do feel a lot better, and instead of walking into town for my shopping, I took the bus, and it was not too bad. However, my son is getting married in two weeks, and I dread the car journey to the church." LARCH was added to the original prescription to give her confidence. Her next report was that she did make the journey by car, and was looking forward to more auto-mobile trips. Her headaches had lessened and she was sleep-ing well. Her last letter said that the headaches had dis-appeared entirely, and that both she and her family were much happier because of her cure.

Girl, age 11. She was in a state of panic because of her school examinations. This in spite of the fact that she was a very bright child, and her parents' assurance that it made no difference whether she passed the examinations or not! She became so terrified that she could not sleep, and when she did she had bad nightmares and woke up screaming. Each morn-ing she had a bad headache and she lost her appetite. It was plain that she was becoming seriously ill. ROCK ROSE the type Remedy was prescribed for her extreme terror. Within four days she was much calmer. She was eating better, and she was sleeping well. After another week, she had returned to normal, and once again she was her happy and cheerful self. She ate and slept well, and she said that she thought the examinations would not be so bad after all. She passed them successfully.

Woman, age 55, unmarried. She was a woman who was frightened of many things. She was terrified of pain, of her condition of health, of death. She found it difficult to make decisions; she hesitated and procrastinated, and wore herself out with nervous stress. Physically, she suffered from con-stipation, flatulence, and heartburn; she vomited frequently. These conditions had lasted over a period of many years, but with the exception of an abdominal prolapse, medical examination and X-rays revealed no abnormality. She maintained that the medicines prescribed gave her "dark, oily, spots before her eyes", and her diet for many years consisted of a small piece of fish, toast and tea. Recently she had suffered from many shocks; there had been several deaths in her family as well as serious illnesses among her friends. It was our opinion that fear was at the bottom of her troubles, and the cause of her physical condition. ROCK ROSE was prescribed as the type Remedy for her terrors; STAR OF BETHLEHEM for the shocks she had suffered. The Remedies, she said, gave her no ill effects, and she had not vomited since she started to take them. Although the constipation persisted, her stomach felt better, and the heartburn had ceased, and in general she was less fearful. She took the Remedies for another three months. All her fears had subsided, and the constipation was almost relieved.

Woman, age 60, a widow. She was a very nervous type, with deep-rooted fears which resulted in frightening nightmares from which she would awaken screaming. She had this state of terror for more than thirty-three years. When her husband was alive, he would speak to her, and calm her down; but now that she was alone, she dreaded these night terrors. Recently she had suffered from phlebitis and general fatigue. ROCK ROSE was prescribed for her terrors; HORNBEAM to give her strength. Within a month she wrote to say: "I am very pleased with myself. I have not screamed in my sleep since taking the medicine. My legs do not ache now, and I can work in the garden without becoming tired. I am so much happier." Later she wrote to say that she had no recurrence of her troubles.

Woman, age 74, married. She was filled with fears. She feared that she might become dependent on others, or that she might lose her husband. She feared accidents when she read about them in the newspaper, and she thought that she would never get well again. When she came to us she was suffering from a skin irritation and pruritis. She stated that normally she was a cheerful and happy woman, and that she tried to keep her anxieties to herself. ROCK ROSE was prescribed for her terror; AGRIMONY the type Remedy because she tried to keep her fears to herself. She reported within one month that she was sleeping well, and that the skin irritation was better. She continued to take the same Remedies for the next two months, when she said that except for two minor setbacks, she had improved greatly, physically and emotionally. GENTIAN was added to the next prescription to neutralize the discouragement at the setbacks. After another month, she reported that she was completely cured, and that she had never felt better, physically or mentally.

Girl, age 10. When we were called in, she was in a semicoma from pneumonia; she had a high temperature, and was very restless. Her parents were in a state of panic, and the family physician was in attendance. She and her parents were given ROCK ROSE immediately. This was to neutralize her serious condition, and to counteract the terror which was communicated to her by the panic and fear of her parents. Her lips and gums were moistened at intervals with ROCK ROSE Remedy. Within two hours, the temperature had taken a sharp drop, and throughout the night she was given doses of ROCK ROSE at hourly intervals. She awoke the next day, and though her temperature was normal, she was still very weak and fretful. CENTUARY, for those who can make little effort because of weakness, and CHICORY, for those who are fretful, was added to ROCK ROSE. Her progress was steady and excellent, and in a short time she was well again.

CHAPTER 28

ROCK WATER

Keywords: Self-repression; self-denial; self-martyrdom

IT is interesting to speculate why Dr. Bach was led to
choose water as one of the thirty-eight Remedies, when
the other thirty-seven were made from plants or trees!
Probably he recognized the state of mind which this
Remedy relieves as one of great inflexibility, in a sense,
as hard as a rock. Such a state of mind has need of the
gentle drops of water which can in fact wear away the
hardest stone! Dr. Bach himself said this Remedy was
for those with strong opinions about religion, politics,
or reform; it is for those who allow their minds and
lives to be ruled by their cherished theories. The ROCK
WATER type are hard masters on themselves. They are
strict in their way of living, they have formed high
ideals from which they cannot be deflected, and they
force themselves to live up to them. They practice
self-denial and they undergo a form of self-martyrdom
in order to maintain the standard of conduct or the
state of health they consider to be correct, or even
saintly. This is *not* self-mastery, for true self-mastery
comes through forgetting the self, not concentrating
upon it. It is a form of self-domination; they rule
themselves with an iron hand. They cannot understand that such practices as diets are the result, not the
cause of spiritual growth! The ROCK WATER type is the
opposite of the VINE type, for the latter try to dominate

other people, while the ROCK WATER folk do not interfere, as a rule, in the lives of others. Actually, this is
because they are far too concerned with their own
perfection, and the setting of a perfect example for all
to behold. It was said about a ROCK WATER person:
"She holds herself very upright, she 'holds herself in'
and tries all the time to be so good and to influence
other people around her through her own attitude and
example." Another said about himself: "I study and I
am very strict in my diet. I don't eat meat, but I eat
plenty of fruit. I don't drink tea or coffee. I neither eat
white bread nor pastries. I live a clean life. I don't
smoke or use alcohol." Let it be remarked that his
rigidity of outlook caused him much more suffering
than a piece of white bread would have done! They
are the "hairshirt" people, the fakirs who mortify the
flesh, the martyrs who deny themselves even the simple
pleasures of life lest they violate the rigid code they
have set for themselves. One wrote: "Do you not
believe the ancient sage's advice 'Thou shalt plant
the mallow but thou shalt not eat its fruit'? That is to
say we should be mild and forgiving toward others, but
not to ourselves." In reply to *that* question, our answer
is an emphatic NO. We cannot live in a state of unfor-
giveness, or worse, unforgivingness, not even to ourselves. We are children of love, and to love is to forgive;
only those who have learned how to forgive themselves
can truly forgive others!

The positive aspects are seen in those persons who
have high ideals, but when they are convinced of a
higher or a better truth, are willing to forsake their
original theories and beliefs. Such people have flexible
minds. They are not easily influenced by others, because they know in advance that they will be shown
greater and deeper truths. The joy and peace that they

experience in life encourages others to follow their path.

Case Histories

Woman, age 70, a widow. She was very strict with herself and had established a rigid pattern of life; she seemed unable to see any other point of view. She was a daydreamer and a fanatic. Since her husband's death, she worked as a typist at home, but chilblains, summer and winter, impeded her efficiency. Her feet were also affected, and at night she suffered severe cramps which often wakened her. ROCK WATER the type Remedy was prescribed together with CLEMATIS for her dreamy state. Within four weeks, she reported that although the cold weather had set in, the chilblains had almost disappeared from both hands and feet; she had some cramps on occasions, but they were not as severe as before. She said that she felt more relaxed in mind and body. She took the Remedies for six months, and wrote to say: "I have worked in an unheated house during all the winter months, and without gloves during this last cold spell. The chilblains have not returned, and I have not had any more cramps at night. I am so grateful to be free from these lifelong troubles! I find too that I am being kinder to myself. I now realize that in the past I have been far too rigid in my outlook and that I neglected the ordinary comforts in life."

Man, age 53, bachelor. He did not drink or smoke and he was fanatical about his diet. He would not eat food that he might have enjoyed, because he feared it would disagree with him. He drove himself unmercifully at his office, and if he could not finish the day's work, he brought it home to complete it. He was always on the go; this, he felt, was the duty that he owed to himself in order to satisfy the high standard he had set. He was intolerant of noisy people, of "litter-bugs", and of what he considered to be stupidity on the part of others. Physically, he suffered from a mild heart trouble, arhythmic tachycardia; he also had insomnia, nervous tension, and indigestion, especially after eating late at night. ROCK WATER the type Remedy was prescribed for his stern self-discipline; BEECH for his intolerance of other people. He felt better after the first month; he was more relaxed, and less driving in his work. He began to enjoy some of the pleasures of life, and to grow in tolerance and understanding. After another three months he was cured. His heart condition had normalized, his digestion improved and he was eating well, and most important, he acted and felt like a human being again.

Woman, age 33, a registered nurse. She was studying to become a visiting nurse. She had formerly worked in the Bahamas, and there she had rheumatoid arthritis in her joints and suffered great pain. When she applied to us for treatment she had improved somewhat, although recently she had suffered from a severe attack. This had occurred while she was visiting her relatives, whom she said had disappointed her greatly; they had not lived up to her ideals. She said that she had always kept a tight rein on herself. She allowed herself few pleasures, and was, as far as she was concerned, a severe taskmaster. She said: "I have discovered that my difficulties are arrogance and pride. I believed that I could journey through life without the help of God or man if I kept to my own ideals of perfection." ROCK WATER, the type Remedy was prescribed for her stern self-discipline; WATER VIOLET for her pride. During her next visit, she said: "The pain in my joints is lessening, and strangely enough, I want to pray and be humble, but I still find it difficult. That depresses me very much." GENTIAN was added to the basic prescription for her discouragement. This helped to a certain extent; when she came again, she said: "I find myself in very real conflict with what my instructors tell me to learn, as I believe they are wrong. I feel so panic-stricken that I doubt whether I will be able to finish the course. I feel angry, and resentful too." Another prescription was given consisting of the following Remedies: ROCK WATER; WATER VIOLET; plus ROCK ROSE for panic and WILLOW for resentment. She took these Remedies for three

months. When she wrote to us after that time, she said that
she had finished her course, and was now working as a
visiting nurse. She said: "My life has changed so much
since I first took the Remedies. I am getting stronger every
day. If I had not experienced the effect of the Remedies, I
could not believe it! They took my pain, and turned it
into joy."

Woman, middle age. She was a strict self-disciplinarian
and very hard on herself. She said that she had suffered
from constipation ever since she was three years old, and
that since that time she had never had a normal movement
without a purgative. Emotionally, she suffered from fears of
unknown origin, and from indecision. ROCK WATER the type
Remedy was prescribed for her strict self-discipline;
SCLERANTHUS for her indecision; ASPEN for the fears of
unknown origin. Within three weeks she reported that for
almost the first time in her life, her bowel action was normal,
and that she did not need any laxatives. She also said that
she was free from her fears, and now well able to make up
her mind. She said that she was a very happy person indeed!
Many years later she wrote to say that there had been no
recurrence.

Man age 54. He was a businessman. For the past eighteen
months, he had an increasing pain in his neck, which ran
up the head and over the left ear. An X-ray examination
indicated spondylitis, and he was being treated by an
osteopathic physician. By nature he was active, purposeful,
impatient; he liked and sought quietness. He had very high
ideals, and denied himself many of the joys of life because
he feared that they might impede his spiritual progress. He
likened himself to a bull, standing with his head down and
ready to defend the high principles he had set for himself.
He applied this idealism to his business and took his responsibilities seriously. ROCK WATER was prescribed for his self-
discipline; IMPATIENS for his naturally impatient nature;
ELM because he took his business responsibilities too seriously.
Improvement was slow, but after two months he said that
the stiffness in his neck had become less, and his wife later

wrote: "My husband can now laugh when he is home." He continued the treatment for several months more, and the stiff neck gradually began to loosen. During this period, he faced a crisis in his business, and this caused an immediate return of the pain and stiffness, and he felt panicky. ROCK ROSE was added to the prescription for the feeling of panic; STAR OF BETHLEHEM for the shock. During another interview, he said that he thought it was pride which caused his pain, for he prided himself on his ideals and way of life, as well as on his work. WATER VIOLET was added to the original prescription of ROCK WATER, IMPATIENS and ELM. After another period of time, he wrote to say that he felt the progress was gentle but certain. He said that in spite of doing heavy gardening work, the neck and the shoulder did not trouble him any more, and he added: "I wish that I could have a quiet life in the country. I no longer have the ambition to be a successful businessman, but I want to enjoy my life and my home." His neck had become entirely free from any stiffness, and his wife wrote to say that he was a different man. He was gentle, kind, and no longer impatient. He was in fact taking life much more easily than before, and he had even modified his impossibly high ideals!

Woman, middle age, married with three children. She said of herself: "I follow a life of self-discipline and the development of the Inner Life, which is my real self." Her medical history was long and complex. She suffered from indigestion; she would suddenly develop a terrible pain in the stomach. The last attack had lasted for ten weeks. Her physicians could discover no pathological reason for the pain, and could only give her drugs to relieve it. The pain kept returning periodically, and although she had seen several specialists, they too were unable to help her, although they did suggest that she learn to live with it. She had a very active nature, and the drive of the perfectionist; yet she could sit in a chair and fall asleep in the presence of other people. ROCK WATER was prescribed for the harshness she displayed toward herself; VERVAIN because she forced herself to keep going; CLEMATIS for her uncontrollable sleepiness, which in fact was an escape from her difficulties. She continued the treatment for many months. The pain gradually lessened in both intensity and frequency. She wrote: "It is a tremendous relief not to be so sleepy, and to be more free of the pain." She took the Remedies for over a year, when she wrote again to say: "My digestive condition has improved enormously. I have been without pain all of the time, and the other symptoms are not so severe. I have become much less tense, and I do not try to work as hard as I did, or to put so much into what I do." Finally, after another half a year, she wrote: "I am entirely well in every way, and I am so grateful! The pains have never returned!"

Woman age 70. She was suffering from kidney stones, and an operation had been recommended. When she came to see us, she was having much pain from time to time, and she was waiting for a bed in the hospital. By nature, she was a gentle, independent person who exemplified the highest ideals and who tried to perfect her character so that others might profit by her example. ROCK WATER was prescribed for her rather stern attitude toward herself; CRAB APPLE to cleanse the body from the kidney stones. Almost immediately after she started to take the Remedies, the pain stopped. She continued to take the Remedies until she went into the hospital. The operation was most successful and her general health improved greatly. She became much more lenient with herself, and enjoyed a fuller, more happy life than she ever had before.

CHAPTER 29

SCLERANTHUS

Keywords: Uncertainty; indecision; hesitancy; unbalance

SCLERANTHUS is the Remedy for those people who suffer from indecision. They lack the ability to make up their minds, and thus they are swayed between two things or possibilities. The SCLERANTHUS type also experiences extremes of joy or sadness, energy or apathy, pessimism or optimism, laughing or crying. To a certain extent, they are unreliable and uncertain, because they are unable to concentrate due to their constantly changing outlook. Their conversation is sometimes erratic, because they tend to jump from one subject to another. In spite of this, they are quiet people, and they do not ask the advice of one and all as the CERATO person does. They waste valuable time because they cannot make up their minds, and at times they may lose an opportunity because they cannot reach a decision. In an illness, their symptoms come and go or move about. There is pain first in one place and then in another; the temperature may swing up or down and progress is erratic. The lack of poise and balance of the SCLER-ANTHUS type may cause various kinds of motion sickness, such as air-sickness or sea-sickness. Extracts from patients' letters include such remarks as these: "I have a magpie mind, full of bits and pieces"; or "Mine is a grasshopper mentality, always going from one subject to another in a disconnected fashion"; again, "During the day I am very active and confident but at night I have a complete reversal. I doubt my decisions, and regret certain activities, and this wakes me up or prevents me from going to sleep." A daughter wrote: "My mother has suffered from periodic attacks of asthma since her youth. She seems to go through extremes of great, though non-productive, activity, and complete exhaustion. She finds it difficult to keep a steady mean." Others say: "My moods vary like the restless sea"; "I am riding the clouds when things go well, and depressed when even the most trivial things go wrong." These quotations are typical of the SCLERANTHUS state of mind.

The positive aspects of SCLERANTHUS reflects calmness and determination. Such people are quick to make a decision and prompt in action. They are those who keep their poise and balance under all occasions.

CASE HISTORIES

Man, age 70. He was, by nature, a quiet and kind person. He had suffered from constipation for the last 60 years. He said that it was brought on through indecision, and the resulting worry. Whenever he was called upon to make a decision, either at home or at work, he suffered agonies of irresolution before he could make up his mind. It had taken him three months to reach the decision to come to us for treatment! It was the sudden death of his wife, and the consequent loneliness, that finally prompted him to do so. SCLERANTHUS the type Remedy was prescribed for his indecision; GORSE for his hopelessness; STAR OF BETHLEHEM for the shock the loss of his wife caused. He reported within three weeks that while his constipation had not improved, he was feeling better and more hopeful. Most important of all, he said that he had decided upon the future course of his life. SCLERANTHUS the type Remedy was prescribed alone. After two months, he stated that he was no longer troubled with indecision, nor constipation, and that he felt much more confident than he did before. Some years later he wrote to us and said that he had no relapse, and none of the conditions had returned.

Woman, age 40, a widow. She had just received a proposal of marriage, but she was unable to make up her mind about it. She wrote to us saying: "My mind is in a constant state of conflict. It is continually in a whirl as to which course to take." She wrote further that at times she was sad, and at other times she was cheerful; she was sometimes energetic and some times lethargic. SCLERANTHUS the type Remedy was prescribed for her uncertainty and fluctuating moods; WILD OAT to help her become more definite about her life and her future plans. The results were speedy, and fortuitous. She finally wrote to say that she was now married and happy, and that she no longer suffered from indecision.

Woman, age 51, a widow with two daughters dependent upon her. She worked in a city hospital as a receptionist and although she liked her work, she was finding it increasingly difficult to make decisions. She could not decide whether to quit her job or to remain with the hospital and the uncertainty depressed and discouraged her. Since the age of thirty-nine, she had suffered from attacks of biliousness and vomiting, together with migraine headaches. Such attacks would last for about two days, and the violence of the vomiting exhausted her and caused her to lose weight. The physicians she consulted were unable to do anything to alleviate the attacks and she was told that she would have to put up with them. To add to her troubles, she was passing through the climacteric, and lived in constant fear of a sudden nausea, so much so that she hardly ate any food at all. SCLERANTHUS was the type Remedy, and it was prescribed for her indecision; GENTIAN for her discouraged attitude; MIMULUS for the fear of an attack. At the end of the first month, she said that she had no more nausea, but she did mention the climacteric. WALNUT was added to the original prescription to neutralize the changes in her life that interfered with her activities. After another three months, she reported that she was much better. She had no more bilious attacks; her periods were light and without discomfort, and she had only a few mild headaches. She had decided to remain at the hospital. She continued to take the Remedies for another two months, and then reported that she was cured, and completely free from all of her former symptoms.

Boy, age 12. He told us that he had a "funny feeling" in his stomach. He was a child who lacked confidence in himself, and was continually bored. He did not know what he wanted to do, and he could not make up his mind about anything. SCLERANTHUS was prescribed for his indecision; LARCH for his lack of confidence. For a time he improved, but one morning he again woke up with the pain in his stomach. GENTIAN was added to the former prescription to counteract his discouragement and depression. After taking the Remedies for another month, his mother reported that: "He is now quite well and very stable. He decided to join the Boy Scouts."

Woman, age 40, a widow. After the death of her husband, she was very undecided about her future. She could not make up her mind whether she would move to Cornwall, or remain where she was. She said in her letter: "I am in a muddle." SCLERANTHUS the type Remedy was prescribed. A short time later she wrote to us as follows: "I am curious to know what you prescribed for me. I am feeling much better, but the strange thing is that my mental vision has cleared. I suddenly found that my thoughts had become clearly defined, and it was then that I realized how blurred my thoughts had been for such a long time."

Woman, age 28, unmarried. She was an actress by profession, an only daughter of Italian parentage. She had always found it difficult to make up her mind, and she was continually changing it. She was subject to attacks of depression for no known reason, and she suffered from constipation and diarrhea alternately. SCLERANTHUS was prescribed for her inability to make up her mind; MUSTARD for the depressions of unknown cause. This resulted in some improvement. After the first month she wrote to say that while she was not suffering from any pain, she was suffering from the idea that there *might* be some pain during her next period. She said that she was also troubled by leukorrhea. CRAB APPLE was added to the original prescription as a cleanser. Two months later she wrote to say: "I have had no further pain, and I am putting on weight. Both the colitis and the leukorrhea have stopped. I look like a new woman and I have a much better complexion. I am eating and sleeping well. Most important of all, I am now able to make decisions."

Woman, age 37, married. She wrote to say: "I cannot make decisions. I leave all decisions to the last moment, and then rush at things and am late. I have two sons, and during the war I worked too hard to get enough food for the family, doing the housework, and moving from place to place out of range of the bombs, for the children's sake. Now I lack confidence, and I feel 'out of it' when I am amongst strangers. I do seriously want to get right, and I feel that I am making things difficult for my family as well as for myself, and that I am losing the value of these lovely family years through this dithering and lack of confidence." SCLERANTHUS was prescribed for her indecision; LARCH for her lack of confidence. At first progress was slow. After two months she wrote to say: "I am feeling a lot more stable and a good deal better physically." In that letter she told us that she was a diabetic. CRAB APPLE was added to the original prescription, and the results were excellent. She wrote again: "I have reduced the amount of insulin that I take daily, so things seem to be improving in that direction too." After another two months we again received a letter which said: "I am so much better and brigher and I can make up my mind definitely now. My mother says that she is delighted to see how much better I am in every respect."

CHAPTER 30

STAR OF BETHLEHEM

Keywords: After effect of shock, mental or physical

STAR OF BETHLEHEM is one of the five Remedies included in the Rescue Remedy, and its function is to neutralize shock in any form. Always use it in case of an accident, for whether severe or light, there is invariably a shock connected with an accident. If the shock is neutralized, bodily recuperation is accelerated to a great degree. Sudden sad news, a bad fright, a grievous disappointment, all result in shock as well as unhappiness. Dr. Bach called this Remedy "The comforter and soother of pains and sorrows". Sometimes the effect of mental shock manifests itself almost immediately in the body. There was the case of a previously healthy woman who sat on the cellar steps during a particularly bad bombing raid on London. After the raid, when she tried to get up, she found that she could hardly do so; her hips seemed locked, and her legs would not respond. Her physician told her that the shock she had undergone had caused arthritis in both of her hip-joints. Another woman developed a blinding headache when she was told that her only daughter had been killed in an air-raid. She suffered great distress from headaches for many years until she was finally cured by the Bach Remedies. Another patient, a musician, wrote: "When I look back, I see that nearly all of my illnesses were the result of shock. Certainly the rheumatoid arthritis was! I was accused of breaking an old and valuable Chinese plate, which I did not do. This was such a shock to me that my hands became stiff, and I had to give up my music." Sometimes the effect of shock is repressed, but be sure that it is there; when there has been a shock, there is always an effect! A person who has received a shock may appear calm at the time; but later, weeks, months, or even years afterward, the effect of the shock will become manifest, even though the original incident has been long forgotten. It may reveal itself as a nervous breakdown, a skin disease, a coronary disturbance, or as any one of a number of physical or mental ailments for which no cause can be found. Therefore, when treating a case which does not respond to the Remedies prescribed, it is well to bear STAR OF BETHLEHEM in mind; it might be the catalyst that was lacking! Try to discover, in a most gentle manner, whether the patient has had a severe shock in his or her past life. Try to find out whether there has been recent stress or disappointment. Remember this always: most people have at some time or other suffered from a grievous shock. STAR OF BETHLEHEM will quickly neutralize the effects caused by it!

CASE HISTORIES

Young woman, unmarried. In 1941 she wrote to us saying: "I was in London until the end of last November (1940) when we were bombed continuously. Now I am just beginning to feel the result of the nervous tension during those weeks. My head and neck feel as if they are in an iron band, and the glands of the neck are swollen." STAR OF BETHLEHEM was the Remedy indicated for the delayed shock; VERVAIN for the tension she described in her letter which would not allow her to rest or relax. Six months later, she wrote to say that she was a different person, and that the pains in her head had almost disappeared. The same two Remedies were repeated, and one month later she wrote to say: "The head pains have quite gone, and the glands are normal again. Before I wrote to you the first time, I had my eyes tested because they were getting so bad. The doctor said that there was nothing wrong with them, that it was just nerves. My eyes have now become so strong again that I have no need of glasses. My tongue, which was always coated, is now pink and clear. I am feeling better than I have for years." Later she wrote to tell us that there had been no recurrence after many years.

Woman, middle age, married. She wrote as follows: "I am going through a time of unutterable grief. The one I love best in the world is dying of cancer." STAR OF BETH-LEHEM was prescribed for the shock; CHICORY because we felt that her love and grief *were possessive*, and this state of mind would not help either her friend or her. Shortly after she received the Remedies, she wrote again and said: "It was wonderful. I was able to cry and the feeling of desolation went."

Woman, age 56, a widow. When she came to us for treatment, she was suffering from a series of shocks. Six months previously, her left breast was removed. This was followed by a thrombosis in her left leg. Five weeks after that, her husband died suddenly without warning. Her left arm was swollen and practically useless. She slept badly because her mind was in a turmoil. STAR OF BETHLEHEM was prescribed alone. Two months later she was able to report that she was feeling better; her physical condition was improving, and she could again sleep the whole night through. But she said that she still had sad thoughts which she was unable to dispel no matter how hard she tried. WHITE CHESTNUT was added to counteract the disturbing and recurring thoughts. She took the Remedies for another two months, and the improvement was gradual but sure. She was finally able to write: "I feel so much better. In fact I am a different person. Both my arm and my leg are normal again. I now only take the medicine [Remedies] when I feel I need it." The patient kept in touch with us for four years after that letter, and during that time there was no recurrence.

Woman, age 50, unmarried. Her letter to us said: "I have a problem about mental depressions which come at intervals, and which have been coming on for a number of years. The depressions started when I had a very unhappy personal experience several years ago. It was a great shock to me, and I think I never recovered from it. Now, whenever I have any unhappy ′events or a situation to face, I have another bout of depression accompanied by considerable agitation, nervousness, and jittery feeling. I mull over my symptoms. My thoughts just go round and round in my head, and there does not seem to be much point to existence." STAR OF BETHLEHEM was prescribed for the shock of the unhappy experience years before; WHITE CHESTNUT for the thoughts that milled around in her mind. After two months, she wrote again to say: "I am so grateful. I am feeling better than I have felt for years. It is really wonderful not to have to take any of those powerful drugs I had taken before. I was never able to tolerate any such drugs because of the very unpleasant side-effects which made me physically ill." She took another bottle of the Remedies, and she said that she was delighted to discover that she had no more depressions, and that her mind was quiet.

Man, middle age, a banker by profession. He had recently experienced a big shock over some financial reverses, and had worried about this for some months. He was suffering from what his physician diagnosed as stomach ulcers when his appendix ruptured, and he became critically ill in the hospital when his intestines became paralysed. Medical aid appeared ineffective, and the situation was extremely grave. STAR OF BETHLEHEM was immediately prescribed for the shocks he had undergone; ROCK ROSE for the terror of his illness, doctors, and the hospital. Half an hour after taking the first dose, the atrophied bowel became active, and his life was saved. When this occurred, although he was very weak, he regained much of his sense of humor, and lost the greater part of his fear so that he could make light of his illness. STAR OF BETHLEHEM was again prescribed; OLIVE for his weakened state; AGRIMONY for the mental torture that he kept to himself. His strength returned quickly, and he was discharged from the hospital to convalesce at home. His progress was rapid, and he had fully recovered within a short time.

Woman, age 46, a widow. When she applied to us for treatment, she was suffering from a series of shocks as well as nervous exhaustion and depression. This was her history: Her only daughter, who was living in Portugal, suddenly lost her husband. She returned to live with her family, bringing her two small daughters. Shortly after her daughter's return, the woman's husband died unexpectedly. To add to the current misfortune, her house burned to the ground because of a short-circuit in a radio set, and they were forced to find another house. No sooner were they in the new house, than the mother, the subject of this report, was stricken with a heart attack, and had to remain in bed for two months. During that time, it was discovered that she had thyroid trouble, and an operation was imperative. The operation was a success, and the woman felt better for a while, but again she was brought to bed for the greater part of the day, because of another illness. STAR OF BETHLEHEM was prescribed for the many shocks she had received; OLIVE for the state of exhaustion and depression. Four weeks after she started the treatment, she said that she felt stronger, and that she could get up from bed and dress herself. Each day she grew progressively better, and she could remain up for longer periods. After another month, she felt that she was growing much stronger; she could go for short walks, she was sleeping well, and was without depressions. She continued to take the Remedies for another month at which time she said that she felt better than ever before, and that her bitter experiences were now things of the past.

Man, age 70, a widower. A few weeks before he came to us for treatment, his wife died suddenly and unexpectedly, and the shock was very great. He had become depressed, and he felt that life held nothing more for him. STAR OF

BETHLEHEM was prescribed for the shock; GORSE for his great hopelessness. Two weeks later he wrote saying that there had been no improvement, and adding the fact that he had suffered from constipation for more than sixty years. MUSTARD was then added to the original prescription to neutralize the black depressions and gloom. Six weeks later, he wrote to say that the depressions had vanished, and that he had regained his peace of mind. He added that much to his astonishment and gratitude, the constipation which had troubled him for so long was very much better, and hardly troubled him at all!

CHAPTER 31

SWEET CHESTNUT

Keywords: Extreme mental anguish; hopelessness; despair

DR. BACH wrote thus about SWEET CHESTNUT: "It is the one [Remedy] for that terrible, that appalling mental despair when it seems the very soul itself is suffering destruction. [It is] the hopeless despair of those who feel they have reached the limit of their endurance." This is mental torture in the extreme. The mind has reached the point where it feels that it can bear no more. It has resisted the stress to the utmost; now all is a void, both in the past and in the future. For the mind and the body, exhaustion and loneliness is total. One patient described this condition in a letter: "I think I know (though I am not very brave physically) what it means to be driven into a world where sight is not seeing and sound is not hearing, and where the closest person is millions of miles away; where even death cannot come to one's aid." The SWEET CHESTNUT type are persons of strong character. They do not tend toward suicide as the CHERRY PLUM type do. They have full control of their emotions, and they keep their distress to themselves. In this regard they are similar to the AGRIMONY people, who also keep their troubles to themselves, but the distress of the SWEET CHESTNUT type is by far the greater. The hopelessness suffered by the SWEET CHESTNUT people is more acute than that suffered by the GORSE type; the SWEET CHESTNUT persons suffer with an intensity that almost seems beyond human capacity to bear. Those who experience this terrible despair and who stand up under it often feel that they must crack even against their will or intention. One patient who had suffered mental anguish for many years wrote: "I feel that I have come to the end of everything. I feel that I am no longer worthy even to pray; the future is complete darkness. I have no hope, no peace. I am in a complete void, I am so alone."

The positive aspect is seen in those who, even though their anguish is so great as to seem unbearable, can call on their Father for help, and still put their trust in Him. Then, as Dr. Bach said, "the cry for help is heard and it is the moment when miracles are done." Those who have ever experienced this form of suffering have the understanding and the desire to help all others in despair.

CASE HISTORIES

Man age 70, a widower. His life had been most difficult for the last forty years; it was filled with disappointments, shocks and sorrows, all of which he had borne with fortitude and without despair. But when his wife died, he felt that he could no longer withstand the stress of life, and that he had reached the end of his endurance. He had become desperate, depressed, lonely and hopeless. He felt that there was nothing left for him to hold on to. When he came to us, his physical health was good except for chronic constipation which forced him to take a laxative every day. SWEET CHESTNUST the type Remedy was prescribed for the depression and hopelessness. After one month his report was encouraging. He said: "The depression is lifting, I am grateful to say. I can see daylight ahead, and my faith is returning." He continued to take SWEET CHESTNUT for another two months. He wrote again saying: "The hopeless depression has quite gone and the constipation has improved beyond measure. I no longer need to take laxatives. Above all, I have gained a true peace of mind."

Woman age 56, married. She had married when she was very young, and quite without any knowledge of sex or conjugal relations. She had three babies in rapid succession, and then practised birth control. However, someone told her that this practice was akin to murder, and she became very troubled in her own mind as her guilty feelings increased. She was never able to liberate herself from the feeling of guilt, and all the time she felt that she would never be forgiven. When she came to us, she was suffering from insomnia and terrifying nightmares. She feared that at times she would lose all control of herself and harm somebody, and she would not allow her youngest child to sleep in her bed for that reason. She was a desperately unhappy woman who felt she had come to the end of her rope, and that she could not bear the strain much longer. She saw no help for her plight. She could see no peace, no hope, no future; just the despairing blackness of the great unknown. SWEET CHESTNUT the type Remedy was prescribed for her great despair; CHERRY PLUM for the lack of emotional control. Her improvement was gradual. After two months, she could say that the feelings of violence were abating, and that she was sleeping slightly better, but she was still filled with self-reproach and the idea that she would never be forgiven. PINE was added to the original prescription to neutralize that state of mind. After another two months, she wrote to say that she was feeling ever so much better and that she had begun to have hope again. Two months later she wrote again to say: "I have felt better this month than I have for years." Treatment was continued for some months more, and no relapse has ever been reported.

Man, age 70, a widower. When he came to see us, he related the series of misfortunes which had made his life miserable for many years. His two sons had been killed in the war. Recently his wife and his oldest friend had died within weeks of each other. He was alone, and he felt that there was nothing to live for. He said that he lacked friends and affection since his wife had died. He felt that even God had forsaken him, and he did not think that he could endure the mental anguish much longer. SWEET CHESTNUT the type Remedy was prescribed for his feeling of despair and mental anguish. His reaction to the treatment was slow, but certain; gradually he began to see a little light, a thin ray of hope. At this point, fate took a hand in the appearance of a little stray dog which he took in and cared for. This was the turning point. Some months later he wrote that he had regained his faith in God, and that he was able to face the future boldly.

Man, age 26, an army sergeant. During the war he had served most of the time in North Africa. He was a fine, strong and sensitive man who was much liked by his men. He had been wounded three times, and was often decorated for bravery. When he was demobilized, in 1946, he began to feel a reaction from the many terrible experiences he and his men had gone through in the war. He could not erase from his memory the sights of the battlefields where he had fought. He started to have terrifying nightmares, and would wake up shaking with fear and screaming aloud. He withdrew into himself and began to shun the company of other people. He said that he felt he was alone in the darkness where there was no light, no joy, nothing in fact but a terrible anguish of his soul, and sorrow. He said that he did not know for how long he could continue to remain sane, and that he felt God had deserted him. In spite of this, he had to work, because he had a wife and family to support. SWEET CHESTNUT was prescribed for his mental anguish; ROCK ROSE for his terror. Gradually, as the weeks passed, he began to regain his courage and a faint hope. The progress was slow, but sure, and he persevered until he was once again his old calm and courageous self, and the memories of the past had faded away. Twenty-three years have passed since then, and he has never had a relapse, nor any further trouble. Today he is a fit and happy man.

Woman, age 63, unmarried. Her childhood had been unhappy, and all of her life difficult. One of her parents had committed suicide, and her early years had been those of stress, poverty and unhappiness. She was a professional musician, and an artistic and highly sensitive person. When she came to us, she said that she lived with a friend who was always ill, and a very difficult person at best. She was starting to have severe depressions, and she was afraid that she would not be able to carry on with her work. The depressions had increased as her health deteriorated, and now she was on the verge of collapse. As she said, she had nothing to look forward to; the depressions were becoming unbearable and there was nothing but darkness all about her. There was no help or relief in sight. SWEET CHESTNUT was prescribed for her hopelessness and despair; OLIVE to strengthen her mind and body. Although the response was slow, she began to play the piano again, and this led to the hope that she would be able to regain her happiness once more. Her strength gradually returned, until finally she was able to accept a few pupils. The depressions were becoming less severe and less frequent. She took the Remedies for over a year, and finally she was cured. She wrote: "How worth while was the struggle to get well! I am busy again with my music which I love. I am playing at concerts again! My friend has gone into a hospital where she will have all the attention she needs."

Woman, age 66, married. Throughout most of her life she was a normally cheerful person who enjoyed life. However, for the past four months she had been suffering from a painfully afflicted throat and tongue. The throat was continually sore and the tongue was dry with tiny white spots on its surface. She herself was fully convinced that she had cancer, and she refused to believe the assurances of her physician to the contrary. She was overwhelmed by a black despair which she could not get rid of. It was fast becoming unendurable, and she was beginning to feel that she would be unable to bear the stress for much longer. She had told her husband nothing about all of this, and she was trying to bear her misery alone. When we first saw her, she had about lost all hope. SWEET CHESTNUT was prescribed for the black depression and despair; STAR OF BETHLEHEM for the shock the thought of having cancer produced. After the first month, she reported that she had been lifted out of the black despair into a more calm and happy state of mind, as she said: "much to my surprise and gratitude." Her tongue had improved, and was almost cleared, while her throat was no longer sore. During the next interview she had with us, she said: "I must not make my illness my dominant thought, otherwise my trouble will become the god of my mind. I have too much of a tendency to dwell in the past." HONEYSUCKLE was added to the next prescription to combat the tendency to live in the past. She continued the treatment for the next six months. There were occasional setbacks, but they were of a minor nature, and became less frequent as time went on. Finally, she was able to report: "I am progressing right ahead now. My throat is well and my tongue is clear, and now, of course, I know that it was not cancer after all."

CHAPTER 32

VERVAIN

Keywords: Strain; stress; tension; over-enthusiasm

VERVAIN is the Remedy for the extremes of mental energy which manifest themselves in over-effort, stress and tension. It is for those persons who force themselves by pure effort of will to do things that are beyond their physical strength. Such people "live on their nerves" and this results in physical exhaustion, illness, and nervous breakdowns. The VERVAIN type hold very strong opinions and ideas which they hardly ever change, and which they wish to impose upon others. They will "run a thing to death" if they believe that it is right. Such are the fanatics, the reformers, the converts and the martyrs for a cause. They possess great courage, and face danger willingly to defend their principles. They are, as a rule, quick in speech and movement, and wiry in body. Often others are carried along by their enthusiasm, and those who are, often become tired and exhausted by the pressure of their influence. The VERVAIN folk are high-strung; they fret and fuss when they cannot do all they want to do. When they feel that they are not getting along fast enough, they are driven to even greater efforts. A typical statement is: "My mind is always a couple of jumps ahead of my body. I fall over myself, and my pulse increases immediately." Another writes: "I am in a state of tension and overanxiousness which interferes drastically with my sleep. I find myself taking on far too much, and being without a minute to spare for relaxation. I overtax my strength, and that too keeps me awake at night, or when I do sleep, I am awakened abruptly by worrying thoughts, and my sleep is spoiled." They are so keyed-up that they never can relax mind or body, and this produces great tiredness and strain. It is a wasteful and a wrong use of energy, for it depletes the body of vitality and this in turn causes lowered resistance to disease. One patient wrote: "I know that I am nervous and high-strung. In my youth people said that I moved like 'greased lightning'. I am not in the habit of doubting my judgement, and I have immense faith in the rightness of my view." Dr. Bach wrote of the VERVAIN type: "They have the enthusiasm and the excitement of the possession of great knowledge, and the burning desire to bring all to the same state, but their enthusiasm may hinder their cause. It [VERVAIN] is the Remedy against over-effort. It teaches us that it is by *being* rather than *doing* that great things are accomplished."

The positive side of VERVAIN is seen in the calm, wise man who knows his own mind and who realizes that others also have a right to their opinions. Such a man keeps his mind fluid; he is always ready to listen to others, and to change his opinions when he is convinced of the need to do so.

CASE HISTORIES

From the records of Dr. F. J. Wheeler, M.R.C.S., L.R.C.P. "Man, middle aged, a very tense person, energetic and opinionated. He had a spasm of pain in the left groin for years. The original diagnosis was flatulence, but an X-ray examination revealed a stone in the left kidney. The man refuse to be operated upon. This occurred in February 1933. Between that time and October, when he called upon me as his medical advisor, he had three severe attacks of pain a week. He was unable to remain quiet in his bed because of pain. I gave him AGRIMONY for his mental torture, and IMPATIENS for the tension. These relieved the pain, and he was able to return to work. Five days later, there was a recurrence of the pain, and he was in great distress during the night. This time I added VERVAIN for his tension and his strong will and his determination not to give up. This occurred at 9 a.m.; later I received a note from him which read as follows: About 10.30 a.m. I went to the bathroom to urinate. For a minute nothing came, then with a sharp pain, the stone passed! I will call at your house this evening on my return from work. The man had gone to his work about one and a half hours after taking the VERVAIN. He brought the stone with him, and it weighed about 3 grains. Outside of a slight discomfort for a few days after passing the stone, he has been very well. His last report, in 1951, was that he was fine, and that he had no more trouble".

Woman, age 49, a widow. She was in a continual state of tension. She was over-anxious and given to groundless fears which affected her judgement and interfered with her sleep. She could never find a moment to relax. During the day she appeared to be active and confident, but at night, her apprehension and unreasonable anxiety tortured her greatly. Her life was all work and no play. VERVAIN the type Remedy was prescribed for her overactive nature and the tension it generated; ASPEN for the fear and anxiety that was groundless; WHITE CHESTNUT for her overactive brain and the worried thoughts that disturbed her sleep. Within four weeks she was greatly improved. She was much calmer, and she had only one bad night since she started taking the medicine. Her sleep had become natural and refreshing, and she even found time to relax.

Man, age 52. In his letter to us, he described himself as "a fighter" and an active, but frustrated person. He wrote: "When I worry, I go overboard as I do in all things, and I worry like the devil." He reproached himself severely for certain experiences he had in his youth. This guilty feeling caused him to suffer from continual nervous tension, from a severe stomach disorder, and from hyperacidity and pain. VERVAIN the type Remedy was prescribed for his aggressive, tense nature; PINE for his self-reproach. After taking the Remedies for two months, he was able to report that the gastric pains had gradually subsided and finally disappeared altogether. He added that he had gained a sense of humor, and that he was taking life more easily and actually enjoying it.

Man, middle age. He had lost the sight of one eye in an accident. One morning, while he was reading the newspaper in bed, his sight suddenly dimmed and he became totally blind. When he consulted an eye specialist, he was told that it was possible that his sight might be restored in three months, but he was promised nothing further. Through the urging of friends, he consented to try the Bach Remedies. During his consultation, he pointed out that he was a perfectionist, and that nothing short of perfection would ever suit him. VERVAIN was indicated for his perfectionism, and that was prescribed alone. His sight was completely restored within one week. Since that time he had driven his car, and gone regularly to the motion pictures, but he had a lingering fear that his sight might fail again, and that he would be subjected to the same emotional shock he was subjected to before. STAR OF BETHLEHEM was prescribed alone; this to *prevent* another shock, and to dissipate the *idea* of any shock whatsoever. Several years later he wrote to us to say that there had been no recurrence of the blindness.

Woman, age 74, a widow. She was an active and energetic person both in mind and in body. She was very positive, and she was always ready to convince others that she was right. Since she was twenty years old, she had suffered from migraine headaches. The attacks were severe, and they usually occurred when she wanted to go out to visit with friends. She was over-eager in everything, and resentful of the limitations which the headaches put upon her planned activities. VERVAIN the type Remedy was prescribed for her over-eagerness and her opinionated attitude; WILLOW for her resentment. Her first report, after taking the Remedies for two months, was that she had had but one headache. Her final letter informed us that during the last month she had no headaches and that she found her life had become quieter and more pleasant.

CHAPTER 33

VINE

Keywords: Dominating; inflexible; ambitious

THE VINE people are efficient, certain, strong-willed
and ambitious. They are quick thinkers who can be
depended upon in an emergency to give the correct
orders, and to direct others with confidence. Their
tendency, however, is to use their great gifts to gain
power and to dominate others. They ride roughshod
over the opinions of other people, and they demand and
expect unquestioning obedience. They crave power,
are greedy for authority, and are ruthless in their
methods of obtaining their ends. They never question
the fact that they know better than anyone else, and
they force their will upon one and all. Some typical
extracts from letters about the VINE type say: "She is
efficient and does everything well and expects everyone to do as she says"; "she laid down the law in her
home, and to all of her friends, who in consequence
rarely come to see her." They can be tyrants and dic-
tators, as are the parents who dominate their home
with an iron discipline. They actually seem to enjoy
their power over others, for they are hard and cruel
and without any compassion for those around them.
When they are ill, they are prone to instruct the doctor,
and those who tend them are kept busy trying to follow
their instructions. They seldom argue, because they
are so sure that they are right. The VINE people have
no desire to convert others to their way of thinking.

They simply demand obedience implicitly and without question because they are right. Whenever they cannot gain power over somebody, they quickly lose interest in him, and simply ignore him from then on. The rigid attitude and inflexible will of the VINE type, together with their inherent cruel nature, often manifests in extreme tension. This in turn leads to painful physical complaints such as diseases involving stiffness, high blood pressure, hardening of the arteries and other forms of physical disability.

The fine positive side of the VINE type is seen in the wise, loving and understanding ruler, leader or teacher. Anyone who possesses these qualities, and uses them to guide others, has no need to dominate; he is the one who helps people to know themselves, and to find their path in life. He is the leader who can inspire those around him by his unshakeable confidence and certainty.

CASE HISTORIES

Woman, age 38, married. She wrote: "I am a blood donor and I have rather overdone it. Now I have head pains, and I am very nervous about them; I can no longer wear a hat. I am by nature very determined. I love my husband and my dog, but I rule them with a rod of iron. I get along well with people if they see things my way, and when they do things my way." VINE the type Remedy was prescribed for her dominating nature; MIMULUS for the fear and nervousness about the head pains. Two months later she wrote again to say: "I am much better. The head pains have gone and I can once again wear a hat. I am not as aggressive as I was before."

Woman, age 45, married. She was the mother of three children from whom she exacted absolute obedience. She was by nature a capable and determined woman. When she came to us she was suffering from an arthritic knee which prevented her from doing many things that she wanted to do, and that gave her a feeling of frustration and hopelessness. VINE was prescribed for her dominant nature; GORSE for the feeling of frustration and hopelessness. During a period of three months, she gradually began to improve. At the end of that time, she could walk normally and without any pain in her knee although some stiffness remained. She said that she felt much better in herself, and that the entire family was much happier in their home. Treatment was continued for another month, and since that time there has been no relapse.

Man, age 65, married. He was a physician by profession. He was a very determined and forceful man, and an excellent doctor. He insisted that both his patients and his family obey him implicitly, and usually with justification. When we were called, he was suffering from lumbago on the right side, and cramps in the calves of his legs. He had at the same time a severe attack of influenza, and a high fever. His one concern was that he was not able to take care of his patients. VINE the type Remedy was prescribed for his authoritative nature; ELM because he felt he was failing in his responsibility to his patients; ROCK ROSE for the seriousness of his condition and his high temperature. Within two days after he commenced the treatment his temperature was normal, he looked much better, and the lumbago had greatly improved. HORNBEAM was then added to the Remedies to give him strength. Within a week he was able to resume his practice. All pain was gone in his back and legs. His daughter added: "He has become much gentler too!"

Man, age 47, married, in the Colonial Service. He was the father of three children; he exacted immediate obedience not only from them, but from all who worked under him. When he came to us he was in very poor physical condition. He was suffering from an intestinal trouble, caused by impure milk, as well as from piles and an involuntary anal discharge; in Mauritus this condition had been aggravated by amoebic dysentery. He was very much overweight. He said that he did not actually feel ill, but that he had shoulder pains, a dull abdominal pain and the discharge irritated him greatly. VINE the type Remedy was prescribed for his dominating nature; IMPATIENS for his irritability; CRAB APPLE as a cleanser for the discharge. His first report indicated that the abdominal pain was less, and he was sleeping better, but the shoulder pains and the discharge still persisted. He reported again within two months, and said that he was in a happier and more optimistic frame of mind, and that the discharge was lessening. He continued the treatment until finally he could report that he was cured. The discharge had ceased; the abdominal and shoulder pains were gone; he had lost weight, and his nature had become much less severe, and happier, a fact greatly appreciated by his family.

Woman, age 45, a healer by profession. One of her friends had this to say about her: "She tells everybody, from the bishop downwards, on sight just what they should do, where their feelings lie, and what good qualities they lack and should cultivate. She is very trying to her friends and her associates." She had been overworking and had a collapse, and she also suffered from bleeding piles. VINE the type Remedy was prescribed, as drops, and also in a base as an unguent to be applied to the piles after each movement. Her first report indicated that she was feeling better, and that the piles had stopped bleeding although they had not receded. Her second report said that she felt so much better that she was able to return to work. One pile remained, but there was no bleeding. Her final report said that the piles had disappeared, and that she was working hard again. She added that she discovered that now she was seeing the good qualities in other people instead of their faults, and that her friends were delighted.

Woman, married, no children. She was a hard-working woman, but she wanted to dominate everyone, including her husband. She always wanted to do good for everyone, whether they relished it or not. She said that she got along well with people when they saw things her way, and her way was the right way to look at things! When she came to us for treatment, her physical condition was poor. She was subject to many colds, and wearing a hat gave her a headache. VINE the type Remedy was prescribed for her dominating personality; IMPATIENS for the tension and the head pains. After about six weeks, she reported that the headaches had disappeared, and that she could wear a hat once again. She had had no more colds, and felt very well. But, as she said, most important of all: "Do you know, I am not half as aggressive as I was before, and my friends have remarked about it!"

Man, age 69. All of his life he had been known as a good worker, and a person who kept his head in an emergency. He had a strong, determined character, and liked to have things done in his own way. When he was retired he developed rheumatoid arthritis in his back and hips, and the condition became worse after his wife died. When he came to us, he was very depressed and hopeless; he could only see the dark side of life and he was lonely. The pain was so great that he could not hold himself erect. VINE was prescribed for his very determined character; GORSE for his hopelessness; IMPATIENS for his mental and physical tension. He started the treatment in November of 1967. Gradually his outlook on life changed. He became more hopeful and less pessimistic when he found that he was standing straighter, and that the pain was growing less with time. He continued the treatment until July 1968. By that time he could walk three miles with ease, and without any pain. He could do all of his housework, as well as vigorous gardening, without fatigue. He had become bright and cheerful, and he was always ready to help his neighbours with their gardens. The arthritic condition had improved greatly. Although the hip-joints were still somewhat stiff, he was completely free of pain, and it was considered that the arthritis was arrested. He continued to keep in touch with us, and he has reported no relapse.

CHAPTER 34

WALNUT

Keywords: Oversensitive to ideas and influences;
the link-breaker

THE WALNUT type has definite ideals and ambitions in life. Their goals, which they are anxious to obtain, are so important to them that conventions which might impede their fulfilment, are simply ignored. It is only rarely that the WALNUT persons are influnced by others, yet they can be swayed by a stronger or more dominating personality, or a forceful circumstance. A link with the past, a family tie, or force of habit, might hinder and frustrate their own plans, and even change the course of their lives. They need to be free from such bonds in order to fulfil their mission. WALNUT is the link-breaker; it is the Remedy that will free them from just such trammels, and which will protect them from outside influences. Dr. Bach wrote: "WALNUT is the Remedy of advancing stages, teething, puberty, change of life. For the big decisions made during life, such as change of religion, change of occupation, change of country. The Remedy for those who have decided to take a great step forward in life, to break old conventions, to leave old limits and restrictions and start on a new way. This often brings with it physical suffering because of the slight regrets, heart-breakings, at the severance of old ties, old associations, old thoughts. A great spell-breaker, both of things of the past commonly called heredity, and circumstances of the present."

The positive aspect of the WALNUT character is constancy and determination; those who carry out their beliefs and their life's work unaffected by adverse circumstances, or unhindered by either the opinions or the ridicule of others. Such are the pioneers and the inventors. Dr. Bach himself was a good example of the WALNUT type. He forsook all of his old ideas of healing to find out a better way to cure people. He did this in spite of ridicule, lack of encouragement, and advice to the contrary proffered by his old colleagues. He persevered even against the strong influence of his own training and background in medicine.

CASE HISTORIES

Woman, age 50, married. When she came to us, she was passing through the menopause. She was suffering from a uterine discharge, soreness, hot flushes and constipation. She was irritated and depressed, resentful and hopeless, and she felt at loggerheads with everyone. Each month she had severe headaches and bilious attacks. Formerly, she had been a well adjusted, energetic and hard working woman, but now she felt that she could hardly get through the day, and that life was a burden. WALNUT was the Remedy indicated for the radical change of the climacteric; GORSE for the depression. The first three weeks brought about no change in her condition, but towards the end of the first month she noted that the discharge had stopped, and the soreness had lessened. She had neither headaches nor bilious attacks that month. At this interview, she said that she was perhaps overpossessive towards her daughter. She had felt so very lonely since the girl left home. CHICORY was added to the two former Remedies for her overpossessiveness. She reported again one month later. She said that the discharge had stopped altogether and the soreness had disappeared; she felt better in every respect. She continued the treatment for another three months, at which time she said: "I am so very much better and more energetic and far happier and brighter. It is indeed a 'change in life' in its best sense! I can now think only of my daughter's happiness."

Woman, age 45, unmarried. She had been under the domination of a friend for many years, and only recently had she been able to free herself from this association. Since that time she had suffered from constant ill health, and bad fortune. When she came to us for treatment, she was greatly depressed. She had a series of colds, sinus trouble, and a stiffness in her neck. She told us that previously she "had a keen interest in life. Now, everything seemed to go wrong." She had tried many kinds of treatment, but without results. The patient *thought* that she had freed herself from the dominating influence of her friend, but the link was not broken; she was still filled with fear and hatred of her former companion. WALNUT was prescribed to protect her from any unwanted influences, and to help her to achieve the final break; ROCK ROSE for her fear which amounted to terror. Her health began to improve almost immediately; she could recover from the colds quicker, but the stiffness remained in her neck. She slept better, but she would often awake in an acute state of melancholia. MUSTARD was added to the original prescription to neutralize the melancholia. She continued to improve, and hope, as well as an interest in life, returned. It was at this point that she realized she must eliminate both fear and hatred if she wished to be entirely free from the influences of the past. WALNUT, ROCK ROSE, and CENTAURY formed the next combination of Remedies; these were to give her strength and to fortify her determination. She continued to take the Remedies for some months thereafter, until her health was fully restored. What was most important, she felt that she was now free to live her life as she herself had always desired to live it, free from any outside influences.

Woman, age 40, unmarried. She was a businesswoman and she held a responsible position; her character was very strong. In the early part of 1957, she became subject to sudden and severe attacks of Ménière's disease and this interrupted her work. She would become dizzy, and vomit, and she could no longer walk straight. When she called upon us, she was apprehensive and nervous. WALNUT was prescribed for the interference in her life caused by her physical condition; MIMULUS for her fears; SCLERANTHUS to neutralize her dizziness and unsteady walk which indicated an uncertainty in her nature. She was given the medicine, but she decided to take it only when she felt ill, and to discontinue it when she felt well. This was distinctly contrary to the instructions which had been given to her. Consequently, she did improve somewhat, but the symptoms returned in the autumn, when she had frequent though slight attacks. After a further consultation, she decided to take the Remedies according to our instructions, and regularly. The prescription was changed to WALNUT, SCLERANTHUS and OAK, the latter because she had persevered in spite of her disability. MIMULUS was eliminated because she had lost all fear of the attacks. Her condition now improved steadily, and in January of 1960 she wrote to say: "I am happy to tell you that I have had no serious attacks since Christmas 1957. Now I can give you some more good news. The ear noises, which I did not mention to you, and which started some four years ago before the attacks, have stopped. So the hearing is showing improvement too!"

Woman, age 50, married. She was passing through the menopause and was bothered with uncomfortable hot flushes. These interfered with her duties as a social worker in the town where she lived. She told us that she was being influenced unduly by others who counselled her to give up working and take a rest. This she did not want to do, even though the pressure put upon her was strong. WALNUT was prescribed to counteract the pressure from others, as well as for the change in her physical condition which altered the routine of her normal life. (WALNUT is the Remedy to neutralize the effect of any change which interferes with the normal activities of a person's life. Such changes could be caused by teething, adolescence, the menopause or even a new mother-in-law.) After about six weeks, she wrote: "The medicine worked wonders for me. It is like a dream, I am a new person now. I have no more hot flushes."

Woman, age 84, a spiritual healer. She found that she had become so hypersensitive that she was taking on herself the physical conditions of those who came to her for healing. Her own body was growing weaker, and more open to the contagion of others' diseases. She was beginning to feel that her own weakness was so great, and interfered with her healing work to such an extent that she thought she would have to give up her practice. WALNUT was prescribed to protect her from the influences of other people. Within a few weeks, she said that she felt much better, and stronger, and she added that she was no longer subject to the illnesses and diseases of her patients.

Man, age 22. As a child, he had been a prodigy, and had been able to read at the age of four. He had taught history in a big school, but he had to leave because he began to hear voices and to have frightful nightmares. He attributed his condition to the influence of a man he had met some years before. WALNUT was prescribed to free him from the influence the man had upon him, for this was interfering with the work he liked; ROCK ROSE for the terror of the nightmares and the voices. His first report informed us that he was able to relax his whole body; that he could sleep without having any nightmares and that the voices were receding. He continued the treatment for seven months altogether and during this time he made good progress in spite of some minor setbacks. The medicine always included WALNUT, and other Remedies were prescribed according to his state of mind. He finally felt a free man again, and he had completely broken with the man who had caused him the trouble. He was offered an excellent teaching position, and he accepted it.

Woman, age 39, unmarried. She was a career woman. She lived with an aunt who was very domineering and quite unsympathetic toward her profession; in fact she did everything possible to prevent her from working. When she came to us for treatment, she was in very poor health, and had commenced the menopause. She told us that she liked her work, and that she was making steady progress in her job; she was determined not to give it up. However, she found it difficult to withstand her aunt's opposition, which she resented deeply. WALNUT was prescribed to free her from the influence of her aunt; WILLOW for her resentment. She saw us again after about six weeks, and reported good results. She felt calmer, stronger and less resentful toward her aunt, but she was more than ever determined to continue in her chosen profession. After another month, she said that she could stand up against her aunt without allowing it to affect her at all, and that she felt better than she had for many years.

This is an extract from a letter we received from the mother of a child: "My small son was having difficulty cutting his teeth; he was fretful, he slept badly, and he cried often. Nothing that I could do seemed to help him, and then I remembered that Dr. Bach said WALNUT helps in 'any advancing stage of life' and that teething was one of those stages. I gave him WALNUT and he began to sleep well and be less fretful and restless almost at once. He is a happy baby again."

CHAPTER 35

WATER VIOLET

Keywords: Pride; aloofness

THE WATER VIOLET people are quite gentle. They are happy to be by themselves because they have great inner peace and serenity. They are self-reliant; they go their own way and do not interfere with the affairs of other persons, but at the same time they will not tolerate any interference in their affairs. They bear their grief and sorrows in silence; they never inflict them upon others. When the WATER VIOLET type are ill, they prefer to be left alone and undisturbed. They are talented and clever, and it is their capabilities and their profound knowledge that causes them to appear proud and aloof. They often feel superior to others, and sometimes they are disdainful and condescending. At such times they are prone to suffer from physical ailments, for pride and mental rigidity often manifest themselves in the body as physical stiffness and tension. WATER VIOLET is different from the HEATHER type, for the latter thrive upon the attention and sympathy of others, with whom they like to discuss their problems and illnesses. The WATER VIOLET person is the exact opposite of the VINE type. The VINE type likes to dominate others, and this is abhorrent to the WATER VIOLET person, who in his great tolerance will never interfere in the affairs of others, although he might strongly disapprove of them.

The positive virtues of the WATER VIOLET type are

found in those who put their great capabilities at the service of others. Dr. Bach wrote about them as follows: "Those who have great gentleness, are tranquil, sympathetic wise practical counsellors, who have poise and dignity and pass gracefully through life."

Case Histories

Woman, aged 60, unmarried. She was the headmistress of a large boarding school for girls. She was a tall woman, gentle and serene, and most distinguished looking. She ran the school efficiently, and she made it a point never to interfere with the staff unless it was absolutely necessary. When she came to us for treatment, she was suffering from severe headaches. She said that she knew the cause lay within herself. For some time now, and quite contrary to her nature, she had become exasperated with a member of the staff, although she had hidden the fact from her. She said to us: "I do reproach myself for being affected this way." WATER VIOLET the type Remedy was prescribed because of the calm and quiet dignity of her nature; PINE for her self-reproach. After taking the Remedies for three weeks she said: "I am definitely more relaxed in the morning, and the headaches are less severe and infrequent now. I can see and understand the difficulties of those who formerly exasperated me." One month later she reported that the headaches had disappeared altogether.

Woman, age 70, a widow. During the years of her professional life, she had held many positions of responsibility; now she was retired, and lived in an apartment in London. She was a very dignified woman who talked and moved quietly and as a rule was not disturbed by anything. She was the very example of wisdom and serenity. Suddenly she noticed that the noise of her near neighbors and of the traffic in the street annoyed her and made her nervous. When she came to us for treatment, she had insomnia and had become very tired and worn out. WATER VIOLET the type Remedy was prescribed; IMPATIENS was added for her annoyance and her impatience with the noise. Within a short time she reported that she was regaining her tolerance once more, and that she was starting to sleep well again. After taking the Remedies for another month, she began to enjoy her London apartment, and was no longer bothered by the noises of a big city.

Man, age 70. By nature he was reserved in his speech, quiet and capable. He was normally patient with other people, but he had become very impatient with himself. When we saw him he was suffering from chronic bronchitis which returned regularly every year in the fall. WATER VIOLET the type Remedy was prescribed because of his quiet, capable and reserved nature; CRAB APPLE as a cleanser of his system; IMPATIENS because of his impatience with himself. He started his treatment in the fall of the year, and he reported a rapid improvement. His chest was clear, and his general health was good. But the next month, while on his vacation, he had an attack of influenza and was confined to bed for two weeks. After he had recovered from that, he sprained his right knee, and it became swollen and painful. He had lost weight and was very depressed. WATER VIOLET the type Remedy was prescribed; CRAB APPLE as a cleanser of mind and body; OLIVE for his weakness and his depression. Four weeks later, he reported remarkable progress. His knee was normal again; his general health had improved, and his depressions were things of the past. One month later he wrote to say: "I am very much better altogether. I have more faith in the Remedies than I have in anything that any physician has ever done for me."

Woman, 51, unmarried. She was a physiotherapist. By nature she was very efficient, quiet, entirely self-reliant, and somewhat aloof. She came to us for treatment because of a large and unpleasant brown wart behind her ear. It disturbed her greatly, and she thought that it might be malignant. She was not fearful of the growth, but she wanted to get rid of it as quickly as possible without an operation. WATER VIOLET her type Remedy was prescribed together with CRAB APPLE to cleanse her mind and body. Within a month after taking the Remedies, she returned to our office to show us that the growth had dried up and disappeared completely.

Woman, age 46, unmarried. She was a calm, quiet and capable woman who liked to be by herself, but who nevertheless had a kind understanding of others. She had nursed her father through a long fatal illness, and during the war she had worked as a censor. When she came to us, she was suffering from a weak heart, and constant breathlessness. She said that one of her sisters had died of tuberculosis, but that she herself had no fear of it. She had many interests, but because she tired so easily, she could not pursue them. WATER VIOLET the type Remedy was prescribed because of her independent, self-reliant nature. The first report indicated that her health was improving rapidly. Her next report stated that she was much stronger, and not nearly as breathless as before. She also mentioned the fact that her sore gums, which she had not told us about before, had cleared up. She continued to take the Remedies for another five months. She then wrote to say that she felt really strong, and filled with vitality. She had had no trouble whatsoever with her heart which was declared to be normal; she was no longer out of breath. She had resumed all of her old interests, and her life was one of joy once again. This occurred in 1951. Eighteen years later, in 1969, we received another letter from her in which she said that she had been in fine health, and that none of her former symptoms had recurred; she was fit and happy.

Woman, age 43, unmarried, a nursing sister by profession. She was a calm, quiet and efficient person by nature. She was an excellent ward supervisor, and well liked by the nurses under her because she treated them with understanding and consideration. Three years before she came to us, she had a bad emotional shock when her fiancé was suddenly killed in an accident. At that time she developed chronic colitis; although she was often in pain, she never allowed it to interfere with her work. WATER VIOLET her type Remedy was prescribed; WHITE CHESTNUT for the ever recurring thoughts that churned in her mind; HONEYSUCKLE for her thoughts which turned to the past. Within a short time, the bowel normalized, and she suffered much less pain. She continued the treatment for another six weeks and then reported that the colitis had entirely disappeared, and that she was enjoying life once more, freed from the unpleasant memories of the past.

Woman, age 70, unmarried. We were summoned when she was suffering a mild, but painful heart attack. During the attack, she was given the Rescue Remedy at frequent intervals. This arrested the attack, and stopped the pain. She was by nature a calm and collected person who moved and spoke quietly, and who made light of her distress. After the attack was over, WATER VIOLET the type Remedy was prescribed because of her calm nature; HORNBEAM was added to give her strength. She had fully recovered within four weeks, much to everyone's surprise! She was up and about; she was able to walk long distances; she had no chest pains, and she was doing her regular work again. She felt her old self once more. But even though she felt well, and her heart was normal, she prudently continued to take the Remedies for another four months. Some years later she wrote to tell us that she was better than ever and that she never had any further heart trouble.

CHAPTER 36

WHITE CHESTNUT

Keywords: Persistent unwanted thoughts; mental
arguments and conversations

MOST of us have experienced times when a worry or
some distressing occurrence preyed upon our mind, and
we were helpless to prevent the thoughts, the arguments, or the words that "we should have said" from
going around and around in our mind like a squirrel on
a wheel! This type of thinking only results in fatigue
and solves nothing. Dr. Bach called this condition "the
gramophone record state of mind". Thoughts go round
and round like a gramophone record when the needle
jumps the groove! As one patient wrote: "I am always
having a mental argument with myself. My mind goes
around and around like a carousel. How I long for it
to stop and be quiet for a while, but it gives me no
peace, and I cannot stop it myself." At times this
mental state can become so acute that it will take a
person's mind right out of the present, so that he does
not hear when he is spoken to. This is a dangerous
condition which can lead to accidents in the street, or
at least to such a lack of concentration that our daily
work suffers. This is true mental torture over which
the sufferer has no control; it also causes insomnia, for
the tortured mind cannot rest. One patient wrote: "I
go to sleep at first, then wake up in the night with a
throbbing head and all of my worries racing around
and around, and I get no more sleep." And another

said: "I get so depressed. Four a.m. to 7 a.m. is the worst time, for then horrid thoughts throng into my mind, and I have no strength to control them." The WHITE CHESTNUT state of mind is quite different from that of CLEMATIS, for the latter type is a daydreamer who is happily building castles in the air, or living in them, in dreams, with a loved one. The CLEMATIS person uses his thoughts to escape from the world, while the WHITE CHESTNUT type would give anything to escape from his thoughts into the world. This over-activity of the mind results in depression and fatigue; there is often a lack of concentration, and a sensation of fullness in the head. One patient found that his "continuous kind of automatic chatter" resulted in headaches for many years, mostly over the frontal area and the eyes, and it seemed to him that "his brain never seemed to cool and clear."

The positive aspect of this Remedy is found in the person who has a quiet and calm mind. Such a person is at peace with himself, and with the whole world. His quietness is undisturbed by outside influences, and in that quietness comes the solution to his problems. He has learned how to control thought and imagination, and how to put them to a constructive use.

CASE HISTORIES

Woman, age 49, married. She had been suffering from a swollen throat for some time, and she had difficulty in swallowing. An X-ray examination revealed that there was no abnormality present, but in spite of this proof she could not calm her mind. She thought about the condition continuously, and had mental arguments with her physician; in her imagination she could only see the terrible consequences of an error in his diagnosis. She could not rid herself of these persistent thoughts, and she lay awake at nights thinking and fearing. WHITE CHESTNUT was prescribed for the thoughts which she could not control; ROCK ROSE was added for the fear that she would not admit. After taking the Remedies for two months, she was able to say that her throat was quite normal again, that she was sleeping well, and that she was no longer harassed by her worrying thoughts. She said: "In fact, I now no longer cross my bridges before I come to them."

Woman, age 53, unmarried. Each morning she woke with a pain between her eyes, and sometimes a sick headache. She worked as a clerk in an office, and she worried about her work at night; her thoughts went around and around in her head, and she could not get to sleep. She was even debating as to whether or not to give up her job, but she was unable to make up her mind. WHITE CHESTNUT was prescribed as the type Remedy for the worrying thoughts that raced out of control; SCLERANTHUS for her indecision. After taking the Remedies for a few weeks, she wrote to say: "I certainly feel quieter in my mind; I wonder whether it is wishful thinking?" GENTIAN was added to the original prescription to neutralize her doubt that she was making progress. Her final report said: "I can definitely say that my thoughts are more under my control, and the pain between the eyes has gone. I have had only one bad headache during the past three months. I am most grateful."

Woman, age 24, unmarried. She had many worries, both over sick relatives and problems connected with her work. She was unable to sleep well because of the thoughts which persisted in going around and around in her head. It seemed as if there were no solutions to her problems. She was very downhearted when she came to us. WHITE CHESTNUT alone was prescribed. The effect was almost immediate. She said it was as if a wall came down between her thoughts and herself; she said that she even tried to put her hand over the wall to pull them back, but she was not able to do so! She had no further trouble, but she kept a bottle of WHITE CHESTNUT always at hand, just in case!

Woman, age 53, unmarried. She was a civil servant who spent most of the day working at her desk. Her job was exacting, and at night she found that she had taken most of her work home with her in her own mind. The result was that she could not sleep well, and she would awaken with a pain over the eyes, and, at times, indigestion. WHITE CHESTNUT was given for her uncontrolled thoughts; OAK because she struggled on in spite of her difficulties. After the first month she was able to write: "I am definitely quieter in my mind and the pain over my eyes is gone." She continued to take the Remedies for another month, when she reported that the pain, as well as the indigestion had gone, and her recurring thoughts were now a thing of the past.

Woman, age 65, unmarried. An X-ray examination, made the year before she came to us, showed a gastric ulcer which had completely healed under treatment. Now, she was worried that the ulcer might return, because she was suffering pain, flatulence and constipation. These worrying thoughts filled her mind, especially at night, and they prevented her from sleeping. She said: "It is like a gramophone record that never ceases." Formerly she was very energetic, but now she tired easily. WHITE CHESTNUT was prescribed for the worrying thoughts; GENTIAN for the depression and hopeless feeling. Within three weeks, she stated that the general discomfort as well as the gas was much less. She continued the treatment and after another month she wrote: "I have no more indigestion or flatulence or constipation. I sleep very well, and I have no more troublesome thoughts. My old energy has returned."

Woman, age 60, married. She wore dentures, and the lower set rubbed against her lip and made it very sore. This kept her awake at night because she feared it might be cancer. She helped to nurse a friend who had just had a breast removed because of a malignant carcinoma. This not only shocked her, but increased her apprehension that she too might have a malignant cancer. She said: "My mind is filled with dark thoughts." WHITE CHESTNUT was prescribed for the recurrent dark thoughts; MIMULUS for the fear of cancer. The lip gave her no trouble while she was taking the Remedies, but while she waited for the second bottle to arrive the lip became sore again. She took the Remedies for another month, when she was able to write: "I have had a marvellous improvement. I have not worried about my lip or about cancer at all. The sore place is entirely healed."

Woman, age 59, a widow. She had just recovered from severe tonsilitis, when she developed phlebitis in her left leg. When we were called in to treat her, she had been in bed for seven days. She felt weak and hopeless. She could not look after her home and her unmarried son. This worried her greatly, and as she said: "Thoughts and ideas come again and again, and I cannot send them away." She held very strict ideas, and she tended to dominate her son. WHITE CHESTNUT was prescribed for the recurring worrying thoughts; VINE because of her dominating nature, HORNBEAM to give her strength. After a month she wrote to say: "I can now go out shopping. The leg has cleared entirely, and I no longer have those worrying thoughts. My general health has greatly improved."

CHAPTER 37

WILD OAT

Keywords: Uncertainty; despondency; dissatisfaction

THE WILD OAT people have a definite character and they are very talented, but they seem to be undecided as to what they should do. Usually they are ambitious, and they may have a general idea as to which course to follow, but the indications are not sufficiently clear, and they are inclined to feel that life is passing them by. This delay in finding their life's work causes them to feel despondent and dissatisfied. They try many things, but none of them seem to bring them happiness. They have the tendency toward drifting into uncongenial environments and occupations, and this only increases their sense of frustration. Here is a typical example of the uncertainty of the WILD OAT type. A young man, 20 years old, was interested in human welfare and in animals but he could not decide upon a career. He worked at many things after leaving school, and finally enlisted in the army. He was soon discharged with a nervous breakdown. He tried to study agriculture, but he quickly dropped that because he could not agree with the methods used on animals. He became a ward orderly in a hospital, and here again he disagreed with the use of medicines and injections, on the ground that they were "contrary to nature". He came to us for help, and by now he was in a very depressed and unhappy state, and doubtful that he would ever find his life's work. After a treatment with

WILD OAT, he decided to start a small market garden of his own. This venture made him both happy and prosperous. Another typical WILD OAT patient wrote: "I know that I can do things well, but I do not know what I want to do. I am in a business that makes me a good living, but I do not like it. I have been in five different businesses. I made money with all of them, but I did not enjoy them. I feel that I am unable to find any business or occupation that I like to do. I am not lazy. I work long hours, often starting at 5 a.m. and as I live alone, I keep house as well. If I knew what occupation to follow, I know that I could do it, and do it well." The indecision of the WILD OAT person differs from that of the SCLERANTHUS type, for the latter cannot decide between one of two things, while the WILD OAT type have so many ideas and ambitions that they are indefinite, and they cannot come to any decision whatsoever. There is an Irish saying that describes the WILD OAT state of mind exactly: "An Irishman never knows what he wants, and won't be happy until he gets it." Dr. Bach wrote about WILD OAT and HOLLY and their special use in deciding what Remedy to prescribe. (See HOLLY, chapter 16, page 107.)

The positive aspect of the WILD OAT type is reflected in those persons who have definite ambitions, and know just what they want to do in life. What is more, they do it too, and they allow nothing to interfere with their purpose. They live lives filled with usefulness and happiness.

CASE HISTORIES

Woman, age 53, a widow. Six months before she came to us for treatment, she had an operation to remove her gall-bladder, and she had felt tired and despondent ever since.

She said that her chief trouble was her inability to decide what she wanted to do. She was in charge of a grocery store, and she was conscientious and thorough in her work, but she had lost interest in it. She felt that she could not be bothered making decisions, so she let others make them for her, and this made her dissatisfied and unhappy. WILD OAT was prescribed for her dissatisfaction and for the lack of a sense of achievement; CENTAURY for the temporary state of allowing others to influence her life. Shortly after she started to take the Remedies, she wrote to say: "I was just called upon to face quite a problem and I am happy to say that I solved it in a satisfactory manner. Also, I have met a singing teacher and a painter, just out of the blue. I feel that there is a purpose behind all this because I am interested in painting and singing." The Remedies were repeated, and within another month the patient was able to write: "I feel much better and stronger; I am much more positive, and I am happy again."

A young married woman who lives in the United States, wrote to us as follows: "About a month ago I felt myself going down and down. I felt so many things amiss with me that it seemed to call for five or six Remedies. Then I remembered WILD OAT and that you had advised me to find my place in life, and when I did, to give myself to it wholeheartedly. So last week I took WILD OAT. The next morning a cold that was beginning to develop suddenly cleared up. My interest in life returned, and I began to feel myself once again. I knew that I must take up the many interests I have outside of my home, and I could feel the wrappings of self-concern falling away, so that I could see and move in the larger world of love."

Woman, age 49, unmarried. She was an American by birth. She wrote a series of letters to us which are paraphrased below. By nature she was confident, courageous, and quick in thought and action. But recently, she said, a complete reversal had taken place. She had lost all confidence in herself; she was haunted by fears, and she had become restless and confused. She started to make mistakes, and to misplace things. She had been discharged from her job, and she felt defeated and very dissatisfied with herself. She was an intelligent woman, and she worked as a lecturer on medical subjects. She told us that the menopause had started two years ago, and now she felt weak, and easily influenced by other people. She also expressed the thought that she had not found her right niche in life. WILD OAT was prescribed for the feeling that she had not found her mission in life; SCLERANTHUS to help her decide about what to do in the future. After she took the Remedies for about six weeks, she wrote again saying: "The remedies worked just beautifully. I am my happy self again and all things have worked out well for me. I am back at work again, and this time I am doing just what I have always loved doing."

Man, age 42. When he came to consult with us, he was very unhappy. He felt frustrated, because instead of following his own inclination in early life, he had submitted to working in the family business. He had a rigid outlook, and this caused stiffness in his physical body. WILD OAT was prescribed for the feeling that he had not found his proper work in life; ROCK WATER for his strictness toward himself. Just after he started the treatment, he was hospitalized with an acute case of hemorrhoids which required an immediate operation. Though he was still in the hospital, he continued to take the Remedies and with rather amazing results. Both the surgeon and the anesthesiologist were surprised at his refusal to take any pain-killing drugs after the operation. Apparently he did not have any need for them, for he was not uncomfortable. While he was in the hospital he made plans to start a new enterprise, and he severed his connections with his old firm. Both his health and his happiness were restored.

Woman, age 40, unmarried. She was a schoolteacher. Recently she had found that she was unable to discipline her pupils, or to concentrate on her work. She said to us that she was in the wrong job. Although she was not sure what she wanted to do, she was a capable person with many possibilities for work. She had recently injured her spine in a bad fall, and she was under the care of an osteopathic physician. He had helped her slightly, but she still had an acute pain in the lower lumbar region. WILD OAT the type Remedy was prescribed because of her inability to discover what her life's work was; OLIVE for her tiredness; CLEMATIS for her inability to concentrate. After two weeks she said that she felt less tired, and the pain in her back had decreased. She continued to take the Remedies for another two months; she said that she felt well again, and had no more pain in her back. Her attitude had changed, and she had accepted a post in another school; she said that she believed that teaching was her life's work after all.

Woman, age 45, a widow. When she came to consult us, she said that her thoughts were in a whirl; there were many things that she wanted to do, but she could not make up her mind which one she preferred. She was about to get married for a second time, but she was undecided as to whether she wanted to go back to being a housewife, or not to marry and do some other work. She said that she had become lethargic about the whole thing; she felt, at times, that she could not be bothered to make the decision which so vitally affected her future. WILD OAT the type Remedy was prescribed alone. She took this for about six weeks, and during this time she decided that she wanted to remarry, and she did so. Some time later she wrote to us saying: "I am very happy. I find that looking after my home and caring for my husband is all that I ever wanted to do in life."

Woman, age 53, unmarried. She was a clever and a talented person who was interested in many things, but mostly in healing, herbalism and painting. She could never decide which of the three she liked best. She became a fully qualified and licensed herbalist and she worked up a good practice, but she seemed to be dissatisfied with that, and changed to another branch of healing. Again she became dissatisfied, and she took up painting. She said: "I am getting on in life, and I must find something that I really want to do, and to stick with it." WILD OAT the type Remedy was given for her indecision. She finally made up her mind that color-healing was what she wanted most to do. She went to Germany to study, and after she was qualified, she returned to England to practice. Now she has found her vocation in life, and she is a very happy person.

CHAPTER 38

WILD ROSE

Keywords: Resignation; apathy

WILD ROSE is the Remedy for those people who have become resigned to their illness, to their uncongenial work, or to their monotonous lives. Although they do not complain, they make little effort to get well, to find other work, or to enjoy the simple pleasures of life. They are the patients who believe the physicians when they are told: "You might as well get used to it, because you have to live with it." Such persons feel that it is their fate to put up with the conditions which are troubling them. They do not realize that the power to alter or eliminate those very conditions lies in their hands! Thus, often they go through life without joy or pleasure. Some typical statements are: "It is no good, I shall never be any different; people just have to take me as I am"; or "I weave things into my life and I take them as a matter of course, and accept them"; or again "I suppose that I must learn to live with it." Very often they believe that because some parent or relative had a certain thing wrong with them, that they too must naturally have inherited it. Such a person is able to say: "It is in the family, so I must expect to suffer also." They are also prone to accept a verdict that a condition is "incurable" and to say: "As I shall have it all of my life, I shall have to bear it." The WILD ROSE type has surrendered to life and to the conditions it has imposed upon them, yet, if they only could realize it, they themselves created those very conditions, and nourish and maintain them! Such persons are always weary; they lack vitality, and they make dull companions. It almost seems as if they have not only willingly given up the struggle, but that they are almost pleased with themselves for having done so! They do not suffer from the depression of the GORSE people, for theirs is a resignation or an apathy.

The positive side of WILD ROSE is seen in those persons who have a lively interest in all happenings, however trivial, both in their own lives, and in the lives of others. Their very interest and vitality attract excellent conditions into their lives, and they enjoy friends, happiness and good health.

CASE HISTORIES

Man, age 40. By nature he was a quiet and reserved person who was inclined to be secretive about himself. Conversation did not interest him, and he made no attempt to pursue it. He said: "I am weary of all that, so why bother to try to talk with others?" He was resigned to his physical condition, but every now and then he would "blow up" and become irritable and tense. During the last twelve months, he had worked in a tannery, but he had developed red spots which appeared first on his elbows then spread over his entire body. He had been hospitalized for three weeks, but there had been no improvement. He then changed his work. He liked his new job, and the skin condition almost cleared, only to return again. The intense irritation kept him awake at night. WILD ROSE the type Remedy was prescribed for his resigned feeling and his "why bother" attitude; CHERRY PLUM for his loss of control over his repressed emotions; IMPATIENS for his irritability; CRAB APPLE to cleanse his system. Within the first month, he reported that he was feeling better and sleeping well once again, and the skin condition was becoming better; he had but one slight "blow up" during that period. After a total of four months, he reported that he was fine in every way, and that the skin irritation had disappeared entirely. He wrote to us again after fourteen months, and said that there had been no recurrence of any of his symptoms.

Woman, age 60, unmarried. By nature, she was a quiet, efficient person who enjoyed her work although she had periods when she felt tired and apathetic. She wrote: "I suppose I must work on, but at times it seems only something that I must do; my usual enthusiasm evaporates. This is not normal for me; I am perfectly fit, I love my work, and I hope to continue for a long while yet." WILD ROSE was prescribed for the feeling of apathy. After one month she wrote again to say that the Remedies had an excellent effect on her. She had lost the apathetic feeling, and she was once again a normal and happy woman. One year later, she wrote again and said that she was fine, and had no further trouble.

Man, middle age, retired. He had been a District Commissioner in Southern Rhodesia, but he was now living in England. He had always felt that he was neither as clever as others in his family, nor was he as tough as his companions. He had become resigned to this negative mental attitude and he made no attempt to overcome this defect. He just gave up. He drifted through life, and left the decisions of his daily life to his wife. Two or three times a year, he was seized with an ague; he ran a temperature, and he was beset with pains and aches. During these attacks, he would just turn his face to the wall and refuse all cooperation. His physician could find no physical reason for these seizures. When he applied to us for treatment, he was suffering from frequent colds, and violent coughing attacks. WILD ROSE the Remedy was prescribed because of his apathetic surrender to conditions imposed upon him; HORNBEAM to give him strength to overcome this resignation. After the first two months' treatment, he indicated good progress. His health had improved, and he had recovered sufficient interest to aid in arranging a pageant in his village. Two months later, he reported that he was free of the attacks of ague, of asthma and of coughing. He had no more colds, and he felt able to face the difficulties in life with a bold front, and much more determination than he had ever shown before.

Youth, age 19. He had suffered from severe acne on his face for over four years. He had been told by his physicians that the acne would disappear when he was older, but instead of disappearing, it became worse. He resigned himself to this disfiguring condition, with the result that he was always fatigued, and that he had lost interest in everything. When he came to us, he was a very unhappy young man. WILD ROSE the type Remedy was prescribed because of his rather hopeless resignation; CRAB APPLE to cleanse his system; MUSTARD to neutralize his dark and gloomy depressions. The Remedies acted rapidly. After six weeks the acne had disappeared, and he was happy and taking much more interest in life. He studied for the National Mechanic's Certificate which he obtained. He became a happy and a successful man.

Man, age 64. Some years before he came to us for treatment, his wife had died from a lingering illness of twelve years' duration. Four and a half years before he had a nervous breakdown from which he never fully recovered, and he was forced to go to bed every afternoon. His physicians could not account for the need of this daily rest because outside of having low blood pressure, he appeared to be healthy in every other respect. He told us that since his wife died he had lost all interest in life, and that from that time on he had made no effort to recover his health. WILD ROSE the type Remedy was prescribed for his apathetic attitude toward his health; HONEYSUCKLE to help eradicate the tie of past memories; OLIVE to aid his condition of mental exhaustion. He continued the treatment for six months. At that time he reported that he felt very well and that he had much more vitality and endurance; he had taken up playing golf again.

Woman, age 54, married. She wrote to us as follows: "I just accept life as it is. I take things lying down, and I will do anything to keep the peace. My husband is a very domineering man and I have no life of my own, nor do I seem to want to make the effort to make one." She suffered from attacks of migraine and vomiting every month; these attacks lasted two or three days, and always left her feeling weak and exhausted. WILD ROSE was prescribed for her resignation; CENTAURY to give her the strength she needed to stand up for herself. The first reaction was that while the headaches remained, she was free from the vomiting. After two months she reported that she had only one headache during that period. After taking the Remedies for four months, she wrote to say that the headaches and the vomiting attacks were things of the past, but most important she said: "The biggest change is a mental one. I have lost that hopeless, dull feeling, and I am able to face up to circumstances. I have joined the Women's Voluntary Service, and I am making friends."

Man, age 39, an artist by profession. For more than a year he had an irritating rash on his hands, arms and legs. The treatments which he had tried were ineffective, and he had resigned himself to the fact that his condition could not be cured. His father had died of cancer at the time the rash appeared; he told us that he had not felt hopeless then, but frustrated and irritated at his fate. Now, he had lost interest in his work even though he liked it greatly, and made his living by it. WILD ROSE was prescribed for his hopeless resignation and lack of interest in his work; CRAB APPLE as a cleanser of mind and body; STAR OF BETHLEHEM because we believed that he had suffered great shock at his father's death. The response to the treatment was rapid. Within four weeks, he wrote: "There was an aggravation at first, but after sixteen days the rash had disappeared entirely. My only anxiety now is that it might return." GENTIAN was added to the original prescription to help him overcome any doubt of his being permanently cured. Two years later he wrote to say: "The skin trouble has never returned since taking your prescription."

CHAPTER 39

WILLOW

Keywords: Resentment; bitterness

WILLOW is the Remedy for those people who look upon life with bitterness, for those people who blame everyone but themselves for whatever misfortune or adversity they experience. Typically, they say: "I have not deserved this misfortune. Why should it happen to me while others get off scot-free?" The WILLOW type feel that they have been singled out by fate either to fail, or to suffer, but never through any fault of their own. They believe that the treatment they received was unjust and they begrudge the good fortune, the good health, the happiness or the success of their fellow men. They suffer from depression, and they are inclined to sulk about their troubles. They are the "wet blankets" who delight in spreading gloom and despair. They have no interest in the affairs of others except to speak with bitterness and unkindness of their better fortunes or to decry their optimism or happiness. The WILLOW people are those who believe that their prayers are unanswered, and their efforts unrewarded; yet they take without giving. They accept all kinds of help as their "right" and so they remain without gratitude and alienate those who would like to help them or to show them kindness. They cannot realize that they alone are responsible for their unhappiness; that they themselves have brought forth manifestations which are the strong substance of their negative thoughts.

When they are sick, they make difficult patients. Nothing seems to please or to satisfy them, and they are loath to admit an improvement in their condition; they often say something like this: "I may look better, but I most certainly don't feel better." At times we all suffer from the WILLOW state of mind. We may lose out tempers and become irritable and depressed, and then find it extremely difficult to "snap out of it". It is the "I'd rather be mad" kind of feeling, and we sulk and grumble and wonder how others can be so cheerful. It is just these moments that WILLOW will neutralize, and so help us to regain our sense of humor and to see things in their normal proportion.

The positive side of the WILLOW character displays great optimism and faith. It is seen in the person who has recognized his responsibilities through the experiences which have come his way. Such a person draws unto himself either the good or the bad according to the nature of his thoughts, and fully realizes that it is within his power to do so.

CASE HISTORIES

Man, age 49, a schoolmaster. During the last five years, he had suffered from psoriasis all over his body. He had not been successful in his work, but he felt that this was due to the lack of understanding on the part of the headmaster and his colleagues on the staff. He said that he had the most difficult class to deal with; the boys were always doing some mischievous thing just to irritate him, and this he resented very much. WILLOW the type Remedy was prescribed for his resentment and blaming of others for his lack of success; CRAB APPLE to free his system of the toxins generated by his negative thoughts. After the first four weeks, he said that his skin was starting to clear up in patches; for the first time in five years he thought there might be some improvement.

He added that he felt very tired, and that now he had returned to the school after the vacation, the improvement probably would not last. The same Remedies were prescribed again, and after another two months, he said that he was forced to admit that improvement was now steady, but that he had some setbacks which discouraged him. GENTIAN was added to neutralize the discouragement and the depression which the setbacks had caused. After another three months, he reported that with the exception of a slight dryness and redness, his skin had entirely cleared up. He said that for some reason he was more content with life, and that he had gained a new outlook that was reflected in his teaching. He, the headmaster, and his colleagues were all happy with his work, and the boys no longer gave him any trouble.

Woman, age 70, a widow. She felt that the blows fate had dealt her were more than she could bear. She told us that her only child, a son, had married against her will, and that she disliked her daughter-in-law intensely. She had been forced to sell her house which she could not maintain without help from her son, and she was now boarding in a bed-sitting room apartment. She said that she had sacrificed everything for her son, and now here she was, left all alone at her age, and forced to struggle for herself. She was not welcome in her son's house, and this she felt was most unjust, and unmerited. She said: "I want my son. I want my home. My son never deserved such a mother and friend as I was to him. He is utterly without gratitude for the sacrifices I made for him." WILLOW the type Remedy was prescribed for the attitude of resentment toward her son; CHICORY for her overpossessive attitude. At the end of three weeks, she said that her distressing depressions had almost gone, and that the last visit to her son's house was much more pleasant. She still resented living alone, and she could not bring herself to like her daughter-in-law. HOLLY was added to the basic Remedies for hatred and jealousy. She took these Remedies for a month. Then she told us that she had softened much in her attitude towards her daughter-in-law.

She had come to the conclusion that she must make the best of things as they were, and that she should not trouble her son by making too many visits to his house. Because of this decision, there was much more harmony and a friendlier atmosphere in the family.

Woman, middle age, a widow. She was a Latvian. During the war she and her young son had escaped to England; the rest of her family and relatives had died in concentration camps. She had found work as a cook in a large household in the country, but she resented the indignity of her situation, because before the war she had been very rich, and she felt that such work demeaned her. She became very unhappy and hopeless, and she was filled with resentment and hatred. When we first saw her, she was in poor physical shape. She felt fatigued and ill most of the time, and her hair was falling out in great patches until she was almost bald. This added to her bitter resentment of her situation and the circumstances which led up to it. WILLOW the type Remedy was prescribed for her deep resentment; HOLLY for her intense hatred; GORSE for the feeling of hopelessness. She took the Remedies for many months; her response was very slow, but eventually both her outlook and her general health began to improve. She found another job, one more suited to her background and interest, and this was the turning point. Her resentment and hatred subsided; her hair began to grow back, at first sparsely, then over her entire head. She told us that she felt much better, and that she was now able to enjoy life once more.

Woman, age 50, married. She had an unreasonable resentment toward her son-in-law whom she thought was neglecting her daughter, and their two children. Recently, she and her husband had moved to another district, and she missed not seeing her old friends. She resented her neighbor who would come to talk with her when she was doing her housework. She had become very depressed; she could neither eat nor sleep, and she looked much older than her years. WILLOW was prescribed for her resentment which we believed to be the sole cause of her difficulties. The results were rapid and successful. Her first report after a few weeks indicated that she was sleeping well and that her appetite had returned; however, she was still filled with resentment. She continued to take the Remedy for another six weeks. At this time she said that all of the resentment had left her. She had talked matters over with her son-in-law, and now she could see that he too had his problems, and in fact she was beginning to sympathize with him! She looked years younger. Her face had filled out, and her eyes sparkled once again. The effect that her emotional improvement had upon her husband was also marked; they were all, once again, a harmonious and happy family.

Woman, middle age, married. She wrote to us the following: "I am full of resentment about my husband's unfaithfulness, and I reproach myself very much for being so. Please help me to get rid of this resentfulness, for all this may be partly my own fault." WILLOW was prescribed for her resentfulness; PINE for her self-reproach. She wrote to us again after two months and said: "I am very happy to report great improvement in my mental attitude. Although the unhappy conditions have lasted for three years, I now can face them calmly."

Man, age 54. He was a bitterly resentful person. He was continually looking backwards to days gone by, and recalling everyone who had caused him trouble. With such, he engaged in mental arguments, and called down the anathema of resentment upon their heads. His physical condition was poor; he suffered from high blood pressure and shortness of breath. WILLOW the type Remedy was prescribed for his resentment; HONEYSUCKLE because his thoughts dwelt in the past. After the first four weeks, the breathing had improved slightly, but then he suffered a discouraging setback. GENTIAN was added to the Remedies to neutralize the discouragement the setback caused. He continued to make progress, but slowly. The first effects were physical; his blood pressure dropped to within almost normal limits and the breathing improved greatly; he was able to sleep better. The resentment about persons and events in the past persisted. It was not until after another four months that he was able to write: "My health is so much better in every way. My blood pressure is normal, as is my breathing. I am grateful, for I have completely lost my resentful feelings."

Woman, age 77. She wrote to us saying: "I have had a misunderstanding with old friends which I have not been able to clear up, and I am suffering from insomnia. I belong to a Christian prayer group, and these old friends and I are the leaders. My friends misconstrued some suggestions that I made, and they said so in front of our group. I am resentful about this, and I am filled with self-pity which I cannot get out of my mind." WILLOW was prescribed for the resentment; CHICORY for the self-pity; WHITE CHESTNUT for the recurring thoughts which kept her awake at night. Within three weeks she wrote again to say that she was most grateful for the Remedies. She said that her resentment toward her old friends had been replaced by an understanding of their attitude; she was sleeping well again. But, most important of all, she had met with her old friends, and they had resolved all of their difficulties. Now the group is working happily together again.

THE COMPOSITE REMEDY

CHAPTER 40

THE COMPOSITE
RESCUE REMEDY

THE RESCUE REMEDY is a composite Remedy which Dr. Bach formulated for use in emergencies. It is not "the 39th Remedy" nor is it a Remedy in itself, properly speaking; it is composed of five Remedies. Nevertheless, because of the lifesaving possibilities inherent in the Rescue Remedy, it is almost an obligation for every practitioner to have some made up and ready for instant use. Dr. Bach himself, and many of his adherents, both lay and professional, made it a practice to carry a small bottle of the Rescue Remedy with them at all times. The Rescue Remedy could well save a life during an emergency when seconds count, and before qualified medical help arrives. To paraphrase a safety slogan current in the United States: "Always have the Rescue Remedy at hand. The life you save may be your own!"

Formula

The five Remedies which compose the Rescue Remedy are:

STAR OF BETHLEHEM, for shock.

ROCK ROSE, for terror and panic.

IMPATIENS, for mental stress and tension.

CHERRY PLUM, for desperation.

CLEMATIS, for the bemused, faraway, out-of-the-body

feeling which often precedes fainting or loss of consciousness.

Preparation of the Rescue Remedy

Add *two drops* from the stock bottles of each of the five Remedies listed above to a *one ounce* (30 cc.) bottle filled with brandy or alcohol; cork well, and label Rescue Remedy.

Dosage

Add three drops of the Rescue Remedy to a tumbler full of water. The patient should sip this frequently, and as he grows calmer, at intervals of fifteen minutes, and then every half-hour according to his condition. If the patient is unable to sip the water, or if he is unconscious, rub in on his lips, on his gums, behind his ears, and on his wrists. If no water is available, use the undiluted Rescue Remedy to moisten the lips, gums or tongue. When used as a medicine, over a longer period, give the usual three drops in a teaspoon of water four times a day. The Rescue Remedy can also be applied to external injuries. It can be used to bathe a painful area; it can also be used as a cold compress or a hot fomentation. Six drops to a pint of water is the usual amount.

Use the Rescue Remedy in *any* emergency, great or small. Use it for a great sorrow, for some sudden bad news. Use it after any accident, whether severe or inconsequential, for after an accident, regardless of its nature, there is always some emotion experienced. The sufferer may experience shock, fear which can amount to terror or panic, desperation with its consequent numbing effect, or confusion. To relieve the victim's fear, and to restore his calm and confidence is of paramount importance to both his present and his future physical well-being. If an accident occurs, give the victim Rescue Remedy; make him as comfortable as possible, keep him warm, and wait for competent medical aid. The Rescue Remedy has no ill effects yet it is quite capable of saving a human life pending the arrival of a qualified physician. In a major emergency, remember that the Rescue Remedy is a potent first-aid measure; it cannot supplant skilled medical treatment and it was not designed to do so.

CASE HISTORIES

Dr. Bach first used the Rescue Remedy, in its original form which consisted of ROCK ROSE, CLEMATIS and IMPATIENS, in 1930; at that time he had not yet discovered the other two Remedies. During a great storm, a small boat laden with tiles was wrecked off the shore of Cromer, where Dr. Bach was living at the time. The crew, of two men, lashed themselves to the mast to avoid being swept overboard from the foundering craft. Due to the tremendous seas, they had to remain in the water many hours before the lifeboat was finally able to rescue them. When it did the younger man was unconscious, blue in the face, and with his clothes stiff with sea salt. Dr. Bach ran into the breakers as he was being carried from the lifeboat, and moistened his lips with the Rescue Remedy. He continued to minister to him as he was carried up the beach to a nearby hotel. The man recovered consciousness before he reached the hotel, and when he was put down there, he asked for a cigarette!

The following letter from a friend in Australia was sent to us at The Dr. Edward Bach Healing Centre: "Last week a bad car smash occurred outside my home. Two people were injured, a young man slumped at the wheel, blood from head to foot, and a young woman sat in the car with a cut in her throat. I ran out with a bottle of Rescue Remedy and squirted it into their throats from the bottle. The man was obviously in deep shock, the woman panicking. I gave first aid, and three doses of the Rescue Remedy before the ambulance arrived. The woman stopped panicking, and the man was calm. At the hospital, they found that the man had a suspected fracture of the jaw, both knees lacerated and other cuts. His head had gone through the windshield, but the doctor did not find him in shock! He allowed the man to go that same night to his own home, which was 1000 miles by train. He wrote to say he had arrived safely and after three days rest, started light work on his farm."

This is another report from a friend of the Bach remedies in Devonshire: "I jammed my thumb between the upper and lower sashes of a stiff window, and I could not release it until the frames were pried apart. It was a great shock, I was in panic and I felt like having hysterics. The pain was very great and the nail had turned black. I dashed for the Rescue Remedy, taking some internally and pouring some into a bowl of water and kept my thumb in it for fifteen minutes. Almost immediately my nerves were calmed and to my amazement, the black discoloration disappeared within half an hour; only soreness remained until the next day. I never even lost my nail."

Another friend from Northumberland reported on this accident: "A little girl three years old was badly frightened when a fragment of a firework went down the back of her neck. A nearby adult smothered the flames and only her hair was singed, with no damage to her scalp. However, she and her rescuer were badly shocked, and the child's screams were out of all proportion to the injury. Both were given the Rescue Remedy, and in a few minutes the little girl was back to the spot where the accident occurred, and was quite ready to watch the rest of the fireworks!"

A friend in Berkshire sent us this letter: "Over the Christmas holidays, I was unlucky enough to dislodge a filling from a tooth which left the nerve exposed. During the following days, until I was able to get to a dentist, I painted the tooth with Rescue Remedy at regular intervals to soothe the exasperating pain. The pain stopped almost instantly, and one application generally lasted for several hours."

Here is a most interesting letter from a friend in Scotland who related an unusual experience and application of the Rescue Remedy. "My friend and I decided to climb the Y-gulley on Crutch Ardrain, a mountain a few miles from Loch Lomond. This is a well-known snow-and-ice climb. The conditions were excellent, the mountain deeply covered with hard snow. The climb up the Y proved to be straightforward, although strenuous due to the amount of step-cutting required. We then chose the right-hand fork which is the more difficult. It lived up to its reputation this time, being chock-full of extremely hard ice, and near vertical in places. As we had been climbing, it had been steadily getting colder, and in fact it was colder than I had ever experienced climbing in Canada. About half-way up the last difficult patch we both became so exhausted that using both hands, we could only lift our ice-axes about nine inches, and we were reduced to scraping feebly at the ice. Since the sun was setting, we were reluctant to stop in such a place, but our state compelled us to. Then I recalled that I had a small bottle of the Rescue Remedy in the breast pocket of my coat. It had been there for the last five months. Carefully turning around, until I was facing out from the mountain, I ground my crampon heel spikes into the ice, and told my companion I had something that we must both take if we were ever to finish the climb. After a good sip myself, I said to my friend: 'Reach up and take a good sip of this.' It was quite a delicate operation since his head was level with my feet. However, we managed it safely. After that we simply remained motionless for twelve minutes. At the end of this time we were both sufficiently recovered to proceed and we were both surprised to find that we completed the last patch in half an hour which was something of a record under those conditions. I am quite certain that we would not have survived the climb had it not been for the Rescue Remedy."

Finally a quotation from a letter received from a friend in Berkshire: "I was cutting a grassy bank and unknowingly disturbed a wasps' nest. They were frightened, and came swarming out and stung me on the right temple, the cheek, and inside the right nostril. I was frightened too, so apologizing hastily to the wasps for disturbing them, I ran indoors and took a dose of the Rescue Remedy, and smeared the ointment* over the stings. All the pain went within two minutes, and instead of having a very swollen face and nose, by the next morning there was no sign of the wasps' stings!"

* The Rescue Remedy is available as an ointment made up in a greaseless homeopathic base.

POSTLUDE

"A glorious view opens before us! We see that true healing can be obtained, not by wrong repelling wrong, but by right replacing wrong, by good replacing evil, by light replacing darkness. We come also to the understanding that we no longer fight disease with disease, that we no longer oppose illness with the products of illness, that we no longer attempt to drive out maladies with such substances that can cause them. On the contrary, we now bring down the opposing virtue which will eliminate the fault."

Edward Bach

BIBLIOGRAPHY

Heal Thyself by Edward Bach, M.B., B.S., D.P.H.
  First published 1931
  Tenth impression 1973

The Twelve Healers by Edward Bach, M.B., B.S., M.R.C.S.,
  L.R.C.P., D.P.H.
  First Published 1933
  Thirteenth impression 1973

The Bach Remedies Repertory by F. J. Wheeler, M.R.C.S.,
  L.R.C.P.
  First published 1952
  Sixth impression 1973

The Medical Discoveries of Edward Bach, Physician by Nora
  Weeks
  First published 1940
  Seventh impression 1969

*The Bach Flower Remedies—Illustrations & Method of
  Preparation* by Nora Weeks and Victor Bullen
  Water colour illustrations by Marjorie Pemberton-Piggott
  First published 1964 Second impression 1973

Published by:
The C. W. Daniel Company Ltd,
1 Church Path, Saffron Walden, Essex, CB10 1JP, England

The Dr. Edward Bach Healing Centre,
Sotwell, Wallingford, Oxon, England
who also publish
The Bach Remedies News Letter (Quarterly)

INDEX